Jamie Wuhn

the Glories of
Sobriety

Inspiring the addict to
passionately desire
a clean and sober life

Essays by

24

long-time recovered
addicts

Conceptualized and Edited by
Faith Strong

Conceptualized Edited	Faith Strong
Associate Editors	Barry Lyerly Joyce Lerner
Book Design	Joyce Lerner

9 8 7 6 5 4 3 2 1

@2009 New Directions for Women

For additional information about New Directions for Women and *The Glories of Sobriety,* please contact:

New Directions for Women
2607 Willo Lane
Costa Mesa, CA 92627

1-800-93-WOMEN (1-800-939-6636)
www.newdirectionsforwomen.org

ISBN 978-0-615-28397-5

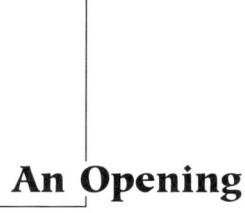

An Opening

About two years ago, a reliable research study indicated that only 12% of alcohol and drug addicts recover. This low percentage stunned me! I began looking for a reason for this deplorable situation. I asked myself two questions: "What is missing?" and "What is needed?" I came up with two words: "sobriety" and "commitment." There is not enough focus, enough sharing on sobriety itself and not enough emphasis on commitment.

I am reminded of a recent revelation during my study group of seventeen newly recovering addicts at a local rehab facility. I was having them visualize their lives ten years from now not having been clean and sober and then to visualize their lives ten years from now having been clean and sober. They had no difficulty with the first visualization (pretty horrible) but only one young woman could visualize her life having been clean and sober for ten years. I was flabbergasted! But, I tried not to show it, just directing them into possibilities. I also tried to have them see that they are creating their futures every moment, one day at a time. However, this process made a huge impact on me.

It seemed clear that there is not enough focus on the glories of sobriety itself. The Glories of Sobriety is not about any form of treatment or recovery. It's not even about how a recovered addict got sober or stays sober. This book is about sobriety, a focus on sobriety itself. What sobriety brings and returns to an addict, what a recovered addict would have missed without it. What it feels like to be sober, free and conscious. This book is about the blessings, the gifts, the glories of sobriety.

Hopefully, this book – with its moving chapters by long time recovered addicts – will motivate the practicing and recovering addict to become passionately committed to a clean and sober life.

—*Faith Strong*

Contents

Take a Deep Breath   7
Harry Abernathy

A Conscious Life   13
Jean Angle

Handful of Diamonds   17
Robert Bush

A Cliff Hanger with
  a Sober Ending   23
Maria Catalano

Following Directions   28
Jane Claypool

Working with Others   37
Debrah Constance
Dr. Gideon Haimovitz

Reflections of Joy   43
Rebecca Flood

A Day at a Time   51
Mary Beth Holtzman

Drunk with the
  Wine of Life   57
Maureen Hoyt

Freedom to be Me   62
Brenda Ives

Sobriety as a Path
  Back to Myself   68
West Leffingwell

Old Enough   75
  Devon Martin

Beauty Lost, Beauty Found   82
  Jessica Overwise

Back Under the Sun   86
  Alexander Popovich

The Avenue of Miracles   98
  Loretta Roth

My Expanding Consciousness 103
  Larry Shrimp

The Gifts of Sobriety   112
  Ruth Stafford

Stay for Another Miracle   118
  Susie Stern

Alive, Awake, and Free   125
  Faith Strong

Getting Out of Yourself   131
  Tom Whelan

Sobriety Runs in the Family 138
  J.L. Wilder and Lyn Wilder

Gratituce and Grace   147
  Loriann Witte

Twelve Steps to Freedom   153
  Rita McCabe (formerly Wyatt)

A Closing   159
  Faith Strong

Take a Deep Breath

Harry Abernathy

"One night a fellow at a party asked me if I wanted a
drink. I was drunk in about twenty minutes. For me,
it was conception. I wasn't born again. I was born
for the first time. I had discovered the missing piece
of my personal puzzle. I was fifteen. I lived to be
forty. And then I died."
—*Anonymous Alcoholic*

That's how it was for me. That's how I remember it. Now.

I couldn't possibly tell you what it was really like. It was
almost twenty-three years ago that I took my last drink at the
old Hilton Hotel in Palm Springs and it was about as seedy as
I was. No, I can't tell you anything important about that.

Remorse and fear in sobriety? I could tell you a few things
about them. But there was so much more to it than that.
Would you understand the thing about me sitting in a chair
for three days straight jacketed by a depression I'd never
experienced before? It was free. A very special gift for someone who had lost almost all contact with his emotions over
the years.

And that should be my segue into what is really on my
mind: the luxurious delight I find, being in my own skin.

Oh, sobriety can be scary alright. Don't mistake me on that.
I'm not going to entertain you with fairy tales. But what a
feeling when the scary part sinks down deep into you and
you really feel what it might be like to be truly alive. To be
conscious and aware. To be willing. Willing to breathe.

I've been told that alcohol (like most other drugs) tends to
affect the central nervous system as a depressant. That makes
perfect sense to me. Life is far too stimulating if you have no

taste for it. I won't pretend that I was chomping at the bit to get out there and take great spoonfuls of life the day I stopped drinking. But, clearly, I'd made a choice. Anything was better than dying and by then I had no other choices. So I took anything.

Living wasn't really something I had planned on. What I mean is, surviving was probably more what I had in mind. I didn't know anything about living but I was pretty adept at surviving. What I expected to be new was surviving without a drink. What I never expected was living.

So every day, for at least the first year or two, there would be a moment when I felt like a deer caught in the headlights. Every day, something would catch me a bit off balance, throw me a curve, or blindside me completely. I had a sponsor and I was attending AA meetings. I was not good about asking others for help but I did it anyway. I sought therapy and discovered some wonderful tools. I kept moving, kept busy. And I learned funny things about myself in the process.

But before I walk away entirely from my former life as a drunken addict, I would like to mention a couple of the things which my drinking and drugging career established on the beachhead of my sobriety. It is critical to my success as a sober human being that I never forget a few odd truths about the difference between now and then. First, they aren't in competition. If I have to prove the value of my sobriety by comparing it to the misery of my inebriation, then I haven't achieved very much at all. Second, I must not denigrate any gifts I discovered in my abuse of alcohol and other chemicals. They are no less valuable for having been found in the junk yard. Perhaps the greatest gift that I can cherish from years of sustained abuse is the palpable intimacy which I have nurtured with my corrupted soul. I have had to stare into the character and personality of someone I never expected to become. And I have had to make treaty with that

8

part of myself, something that most people will never have occasion to undertake.

Finally, as I used to tell my students at a Health Services seminar at the local community college, the patient in recovery has been on a journey. It's a journey unlike any other. No travel agent can book your flight for such a voyage. There are no such trips anywhere in the sober world. That's why we change. We're the fortunate survivors. We aren't looking for the same destinations in our sober life. I believe we must let go of the comparisons if we are truly to be free of the old life.

One of the early things I discovered about myself in sobriety was that I hadn't the first idea of what the word "adult" meant. But I had spent twenty-five years mimicking what I believed an adult looked like. There I was, forty, overweight, prematurely many things and immaturely everything else. Like some prehistoric insect caught in sap, I was stopped at a juvenile stage long gone and over. I had to grow up and it was painful. And it was delightful and rich and rewarding. And it was humiliating and frightening. Yoicks! I was adrift.

Perhaps you are like me and you have noticed that adult people seem to be busy, active, and engaged. It appears to be so dynamic, such a calorie burner to be an adult. That's what I thought anyway. So, I got right into being busy and that got me right into trouble. I got anxious. I got confused. I got behind. I got angry.

Anger? Where the heck did that come from? So I added it to my list of things to attend to. And it was getting pretty long. There was the old marriage which had to go. A different career. A new direction. New location! This was heady stuff, this getting sober.

I banged around like that for about four years. One day a close and dear friend who knew a thing or two said to me, "Harry, you haven't done your First Step." Oh hell, I was way too busy being a poster child for recovery to have to put up with that crap. I was so clean and sober I almost hit him.

I guess you could say that day was when I really began my recovery in earnest. I stopped. Pretty much that sums it up. I just stopped. And I waited for the next right thing to do. Then I did it and then I waited. And then the next thing came along and I did it. I sometimes remind folks who are new to recovery that sober life is often like taking the bus downtown. You get off the A bus and wait to transfer to the B bus which takes you to the corner where you wait for the C bus. The whole time you are making your way downtown. It's just that the waiting at the bus stops seems like you're going nowhere. But it only seems that way. Actually the trip downtown takes a certain amount of waiting. But it doesn't mean you're not moving. The truth is, there's no such thing as not moving. Just ask an astronomer. Every single thing in the universe is in motion, always in motion, never at rest. So relax. Take a breath and sit back. You're going places. Whether you like it or not.

Maybe you'll turn your eye inward and set out on the greatest journey of all. Addictions may be a sickness of the body. They may be a sickness of the brain. In my experience, they most certainly are a sickness of the soul. We all need to go there from time to time. However you do it, that's your own business. But I have met too many sober people who stayed mean, stayed angry, stayed miserable and I wouldn't wish it on anyone. Soul work is where the gifts really come from.

So what are these gifts that I'm so happy to talk about? Why, they're the ones you already have! I'm not suggesting that sobriety is like an Easter Egg hunt. You don't stop drinking so you can start looking for the goodies. Ha! That's just the same old addiction in another form. It isn't your jewelry drawer you're changing. It's your vision.

Take a long look at the Serenity Prayer. If the God stuff both-
ers you, cross it out. If AA troubles you, relax. They didn't
invent it. They just adopted it. Take a look at what it says.
Serenity. Courage. Wisdom. If you had those three things
when you were out there, then obviously you have picked
the wrong chapter. Have you ever had them in your life?
Serenity is necessary so that we can let go of all the people,
places, and things we think that we can (and should) control
(for their own good, of course). Courage, and I mean real
courage, is what it takes to change the myriad aspects of ourselves that get directly in the way of useful goodness. And
just enough Wisdom that we don't get the two confused.
Maybe along the way we pare down the ego enough so that
our noses don't get in the way of other people's businesses.
But that isn't required. It's just that it would be such a nice
change.

Wow! What about health, love, success, happiness, intimacy,
honesty, openness, et al? Well, maybe. If you are fortunate
some things will come your way but there's no guarantee.
Life does go on, whether you stay sober or not. It is messy.

The gift is being okay with it. The gift is learning that this is
enough and that enough is a fortune.

I wish you everything that you could want. And if those
things do not come to pass, I wish you at least the serenity,
courage, and wisdom to know the difference.

Amen.

Biography

Born in 1945, I began drinking and drugging when I was fifteen. Between then and July of 1985, I somehow managed to miss death innumerable times and by as little as several inches. I wreaked havoc in my own life and the lives of many others. I was one unholy mess of a human. My son was my intervention and I decided to try living instead of drinking. Then I went to Betty Ford. I am sixty-three years old and I do believe that I am the most fortunate person alive. Everything else about my life is only statistical anomaly. The best thing about living is the breathing. That's my motto.

Discussion/Reflection Questions

1. How do I handle being loved by friends and family after so many years of despising myself?

2. How do I incorporate other disciplines, such as meditation, into my recovery?

3. How can I be of service to others?

A Conscious Life

Jean Angle

On July 8, 2007, my family, friends, students and AA tribe gave me a party in North Laguna at the home of David Robbins, to celebrate my forty years of sobriety. There were over one hundred people there. The night was magical, the food delicious, the flowers in bloom and the energy transcendent. My wonderful sponsees gave me a thorough roasting. They didn't miss much. In thanking them and defending myself for my brand of "Tough Love," I made it clear that this was a celebration about using the AA Steps to make the unconscious conscious.

Giving up alcohol was only the beginning of a long journey. The end result has been freedom from my addictions and a degree of self-honesty I never dreamed possible. I have been loyal, happy and active in my 12 step programs.

I have been teaching classes on consciousness since 1980. One of them is entitled "Addiction and the Dissatisfied Soul". These Classes help reveal the underlying disorder that causes our addictions. The students uncover hidden addictions to intensity, risk taking, codependence and other behaviors, which do not necessarily involve substance abuse. The solutions to these soul yearnings are often surprising in their simplicity.

In this class we all seem to discover and agree that the deeper underlying disorder of our addictions is depression. As we make these victim, outcast and self-sabotaging aspects of ourselves conscious, the depression lifts. Of course the first requirement is to give up the addiction. Practicing an addiction represses information and feelings and we stay depressed. Since we teach what we need to learn, I have learned a great deal and find myself making wiser life choices.

When I was new in AA, I called my parents in Chicago to tell them. They asked me not to come home and embarrass them by going to "those meetings." That was 1967. A few years later they had read the Big Book and gotten some education on alcoholism, (they didn't drink at all) and invited me home. I noticed at every visit that they were getting more and more depressed. I called their doctor to check their medication. There was no problem. One day the light went on. They weren't getting more depressed. I was getting well.

I have raised five children, two boys and three girls. They are all alcoholics. The fourth child, Alice, died of alcoholism.

Alice got sober when she was twenty-three. She called me and said she was ready to quit drinking. I took her to Seattle where my sponsor, Marion Schoen, ran a rehab center, Residence Twelve. Alice stayed there for seven months and then returned to Laguna Beach and lived with me for another six months. She had a love affair with the program and was very active.

At the end of five glorious happy years, she started using a doctor-prescribed pain medicine. She went into a severe depression and was never able to stay sober again. She spent a great deal of time in Mexico, got married and had a daughter, Mariah. On one of her binges, she went blind. I entered some intensive therapy to see what I was blind to. At the end of six months I discovered that I was blind to the fact that Alice didn't want a teacher, she wanted a mother. When I made this conscious, Alice got her sight back. But she still couldn't stay sober. She blamed me for the relapse. She died when she was forty.

The grief was overwhelming. Nine months after her death, I was suffering a depression. The doctors couldn't seem to find anything wrong so I went to a health center in San Diego where I fasted and drank wheat grass for 3 weeks. I learned a great deal and at the end of the time I found a lump in my breast; it was cancer. I felt there was an interesting connection between Alice's death and my getting cancer nine months later. I do have to admit, the cancer was no big deal. I went for my radiation and surgery and I can't tell you how much support and love I received from my friends, family and teachers. What was a big deal is that I received the grace of forgiveness. For three years, I had harbored resentment at Alice's father and her sponsor and I had found myself unable to forgive. I could only be willing. Then one day during meditation I realized that I had been graced with forgiveness.

Today I am grateful that I had Alice in my life for forty years. She was so much fun and a great teacher. She gave her family a gift with her sacrifice – everyone else stayed sober.

Little did I know at that first AA meeting what lay ahead of me. I had no idea how wondrous freedom from addiction would feel. Today I have happier relationships with friends and family and confidence that the steps will keep me sober. I have the capacity to be honest. I am glad this is my path. More is revealed. The promises have come true. I have moved out of doing into being; I have the opportunity to help a lot of people. I teach classes, write an astrology column and have people who do therapy with me. I also facilitate workshops for my teacher, Brugh Joy. I am grateful to all my teachers. On my next birthday I will be 80. Life is good.

The outstanding glory I received in sobriety is the gift of a conscious life.

Biography

Jean Angle was a periodic, blackout alcoholic. Her disease was delayed due to life style influences. Her parents did not drink – although her grandmother started drinking at seventy and was an immediate alcoholic. Her high school friends did not drink and she attended Northwestern University in Evanston, Illinois, which was dry. She and her husband left the Chicago area and moved to southern California where they had five children and started the first Teflon Company. They were too busy to drink. Around thirty they started to drink socially and Jean started a duplicate bridge center and almost immediately found her drinking progressing from one day binges to eventually weekends and then five day blackouts. She got a divorce and in 1967 attended her first AA meeting and has been clean and sober ever since. Working the steps has been her solution and has also served her in giving up many other addictions. Her children are all sober. For the past twenty-eight years she has been teaching classes in metaphysics and astrology in Laguna Beach, California. She also facilitates study groups for her teacher, Brugh Joy.

Discussion/Reflection Questions

1. What are the most obvious signs that you are flirting with a relapse?

2. What steps can you take to become more conscious?

For Faith, who suggested the possibility that maybe
I could not do this alone.

Handful of Diamonds

Robert Bush

I looked out over the ocean, a beautiful summer day, the sun
sparkling on the water as if God himself had thrown out a
handful of diamonds. I took a sip of a deliciously sinful
cabernet. My six-month old son was in my arms. I had been
to Yale and to jail. I had been in over fifty countries and
painted hundreds of brilliant works. For some unknown reason at that moment I put my glass down. I was drained,
empty and scared. I did not know which way to turn, nor
why. The addict in me was completely defeated. With all my
training and creative intelligence I knew I could not go on. I
needed help. This time I could not do it alone.

With the patient help of friends, AA and the 12 Steps, a
sponsor, a psychiatrist and a lot of willingness to just show
up I began to reshuffle and reconstruct my life. I remember
early on in my sobriety I had a dream which I later painted. I
had been in a terrible accident and was cut into hundreds of
pieces. I found I was in a hospital being intricately sewn up. I
gingerly walked down the hall to a warm room with soft
lights and carefully lay down in bed. I was starting to put
together a new life.

I took actions that were beneficial for me even though I did
not always want to do them. I began to go to AA meetings
and 12 Step meetings and listen. I worked with a sponsor
and did what he suggested. He told me being in the middle
was alright. I had always before lived on the extreme highs
and lows. I rebelled at every turn but kept coming back
because I knew that my way, my ego, had not helped me go
where I needed to go. I started to examine my honesty and

attitudes. I tried to live in the present instead of the future and the past.

Much of my recovery has been felt in retrospect – noticing a different attitude or action. One day I find myself thinking of someone else's best interest or how I can be of help by giving my time or listening to others' problems. Another day I notice I am dancing or silently meditating on nature. Sobriety has brought me an expanding openness to ask questions and a chance to search for my purpose in life.

It has not been an easy road to sobriety and recovery from addiction but it has been a meaningful and rewarding one. I lay beside my father having a wonderful conversation shortly before he passed and held my mother as she took her last breath. I was able to watch my daughter enter this world. I was with my wife at the hospital after she had a car accident. I was able to walk through my open heart surgery and travel to India a few months later. I was present to help my son fight his addiction and to provide the tough unconditional love necessary for his struggle for a successful future, sober, not drunk.

I did not know nor do I know what living sober had in store for me. But I have come to trust that it will lead to a better tomorrow. If you are reading this now, you probably know someone with an addiction issue or you may have an addiction. I can tell you that it will not be easy and it will be painful at times but there is a solution. There is a way to live clean and sober and it probably is the only way to live for you or your loved ones that will ensure a chance for a positive life.

The change for me was profound, as it is simple. It is a change that I must honor and pay attention to every day. Sometimes every hour, minute, second I need to stop, breathe, let go, feel, and then with an intuitive heart make a little step. I need to walk with awareness and run with abandon. I need to care for others while risking the future I believe in. I need to laugh and cry honestly while loving unconditionally. I have to get out of my ego and accept the unknown infinite. I have to walk through the soft darkness into the clear light.

This may sound somewhat abstract. To be more concrete I will share what I have done this year as an instance of what sobriety gives to me. Last year my daughter, at thirteen, said that she wanted to take a year and travel. I listened and the stars lined up and we were off to southern France. She went to a French school. Speaking hardly any French she progressed through the year and as the year came to a close she was fluent in French, had a group of good friends and was at the top of her class. She saw and experienced a different culture than our own and a different way of life.

I was able to spend a great deal of time listening to her concerns and discoveries. We were able to share experiences from the solemnity of a Christmas Eve service at Notre Dame in Paris to the raucous Bear Festival in the Pyrenees near the Spanish border. We went to many concerts and bull fights and toured countless castles and churches. We studied the architecture and landscape of Europe and drew together, everywhere. We went through violent lightning and thunderstorms and looked at the stars. We climbed mountains and swam in the Mediterranean. We saw exhibits in the major museums of Paris discovering new artists and reconnecting with familiar ones. We visited the palace and gardens of Versailles and saw the stained glass windows of Chartres Cathedral. We visited famous cities such as Florence and Venice and we discovered small villages in the Dordogne and wandered in the streets of Arles, St. Remy and Aix-en-Provence. We saw where Van Gogh made the last paintings in his life and where prehistoric men had painted bison and other animals in caves. We watched flocks of sheep grazing and giving birth in the small village where we lived. We shared with French friends and ate new foods. We explored the wonderful outdoor markets. We went to pilgrimage sites and to abbeys hidden in the mountains. We witnessed bulls running in the streets of small towns and went to fairs, movies and art exhibits. We shopped for clothes, and more clothes. We shared music and played cards and read.

Most importantly we spent quality time together, walking out our front door through the stone buildings past the church beyond the chateau to muse on the clouds passing, the color of the yellow and red vines in the fall, pink orchard blossoms in the late winter, red poppies in the early spring, lavender fields in the late spring, sunflowers in the early summer. From playing in the snows in the mountains of the Ardèche to swimming in the rivers in the Cevennes, our childlike exploration was a precious and rare thing. My daughter filled notebooks and diaries with stories of her journeys and feelings and drawings of everything from the Parthenon in Athens to a monastery high above the ocean on the Cycladic Island of Amorgos, Greece. My daughter and I collaborated on a creative sojourn in a small village in southern France last year and in the process we became better friends.

This past year is what sobriety has brought to me – possibilities that become realities, realities that lead to more possibilities. To say what I would have missed if I were not sober is easy – a chance to get a glimpse at the joy of life. I most probably would not be around to witness life if I had not found a way to live sober. I would have died of an overdose, liver disease, driving drunk or any number of the reckless twists and turns that addictive behavior uncontrollably delivers. My addiction clouded, distorted, exaggerated and made my life out of control. It blew up my ego and deflated others I loved. To pick up a drink for me is suicide.

My commitment is simple. It is a commitment a day at a time to never drink. It is a commitment to be ever vigilant to the cunning baffling powers of the mind and body to fool me into thinking that I am not an addict. If I can live a life that is true to myself and honors my family and friends, that lets me walk gently on the planet and be a citizen of the world, that infuses my being with divine mystery and wonder, then I have a chance.

Now, again I look out over the ocean, in Greece or California, and see the same glittering shimmer on the waves. Now I AM that handful of diamonds glistening on the wave, dissolving into the sea.

Today is my twenty-third anniversary of getting sober. I can think of no better way to celebrate than to share my message with you.

Biography

A citizen of the world, Robert Burton Bush was born in Palo Alto, California. Robert is an artist having lived, painted and exhibited in many countries including Brazil, Mexico, Greece, France, Australia, Indonesia, India and the Philippines. Robert has been an arts administrator and development director for arts and environmental groups and women's recovery. He attended elementary and secondary school in the San Francisco bay area and went on to Yale University and to the University of California, Berkeley. Robert is the proud friend to his family, Carolyn, Burton, Rewa and Wendy.

Discussion/Reflection Questions

1. What are you living for?

2. Is there something that you do not know?

3. Are you alone or a part of something larger?

A Cliff Hanger with a Sober Ending

Maria Catalano

Sitting on an upholstered church pew stationed within a five by seven foot cubicle in the old Santa Ana court house on a blustery southern California day recently, a familiar thought blended with the joy filled moment: "If not for the gift of my sobriety I would not be a part of this blessing right now." My seventeen-year-old son, sitting next to my two girlfriends and me, watched, listened, shared in nuptial exchanges between my daughter and "her man," both nineteen years of age. I sure was happy to be one of their four chosen guests.

I am even more grateful for the event that led me through twenty-four years of sobriety to my daughter's happiest day. Thinking back on the first day of my sobriety, everything was as dark as black, my eyes barely opened to mere slits. Suddenly, a bright blinding light was suspended above me. I thought I'd died and gone to heaven.

In the next instant, stark reality pierced my inebriated state. Opening one eye wider, the brassy flash of a police officer's badge became visible. The harsh reality of my absent emotion…I closed my eyes completely to another living nightmare my alcohol abuse had created. The officer's words ring deep within my inner self even now: "You're a beautiful young lady, why would you want to do something like this to yourself? You better think about the people who care about you and straighten yourself out." All I could comprehend at the time was how the officer had an amazing likeness to the TV character Officer Poncherelli from the hit show "Chips" – a handsome, uniformed, caring, community service man.

Then I realized that I couldn't move. His image and voice dimmed and the light went to dark once more.

I awoke to the sounds of a drunk tank. I was in jail and released at first light that same morning. The worst was walking out to see my father's forlorn face. He said very little. The tears in his Sicilian eyes said it all. I was more than a disappointment to him. We went to my mother and father's home – the house where I had been brought up. As I sobered up, reading from a police report my parents reminded me of my drunken escapade. The following day it would be the lead story in the newspapers.

From the newspapers I found out that the bright light I had seen was from the tallest existing county crane at that time. I also discovered that I had flipped my car over a cliff, leaving my life suspended above a two thousand foot drop.

I walked away with a split lip and a badly bruised body on the outside and emptiness inside. These were my first days of sobriety.

My mother had a childhood friend who had been sober for nearly ten years, named Adelle. She took me to my first Alcoholics Anonymous meeting. Adelle was my AA sponsor for ten years – until her time to pass to the Lord's Kingdom.

After finishing a month of court-ordered work, a year of private counseling with a drug and alcohol counselor, and County group counseling – along with daily AA meetings, I managed to stay sober.

However, something was still missing.

One evening at an AA meeting a man who had worked on the Alaskan pipeline spoke. He told of his first days being sober. His doctor had told him his days were numbered – to try AA. So he went to an AA meeting drunk and the Greeter at the door stopped him, opened up a Big Book to the first page. The Greeter instructed him to study it and "Don't drink no matter what and come back tomorrow." Well, somehow he put together the minutes, the hours, and stayed sober and returned the second night. He told the Greeter that he couldn't understand why studying the first page was so important. The Greeter told him to do exactly the same thing. He did and remained sober for 48 hours, a miracle in itself! Although still baffled he returned the third night sober to see the same Greeter at the door of the building where an AA meeting was being held. He told the Greeter he was grateful for his two days of sobriety but felt that the Greeter was crazy, since the first page of the Big Book is blank. The Greeter said, "That's right." The newcomer insisted "But there's nothing on this page!" The Greeter responded: "And that's just about what you know about life and living it...nothing...now you can come in." Summing up, the man ended his talk at the AA meeting: "I start every day with a blank page and let God write my script!"

This "Greeter" story conveys what was missing in my life. Today, God is the centerpiece of my life. In the AA Program I heard it said, "Take what you like and leave the rest." I liked just about everything I heard. I finally found a group I fit into. Wherever I go I am never alone with God in my heart and sober members of Alcoholics Anonymous by my side. I am alive today because I am sober! I have a relationship with God, others and myself because I am sober.

I am the mother of two fantastic children because I am alive living a sober life.

I have walked through adversity – gratefully sober.

When fear, despair, depression and self-hate appear I fall back on the tools of the AA Program, the 12 Steps, the Promises, How it Works.

I also am especially close to Psalms 20 through 25 and a meditation a roommate gave me. I use it during moments when I want to run away...like being in the principal's office with one of my children or divorce court or the Orange County Children's Mental Health Services (asking for funding to help one of my children learn to live a better life). I close my eyes, wrap up my burden, trouble, or problem in a beautiful package; then a condor swoops down and carries it into a fountain of fire.

I continue to learn being sober. I remain open to others being sober. I can accept, surrender and find joy being sober.

When my nineteen-year-old daughter told me she was getting married in a week, I accepted it with blessings. Because of my love for her I had no other choice. Being sober gives me such choices.

When Faith Strong asked me to write this chapter I was full of fear. If it weren't for my sobriety I would not be writing this essay for you now. I remember every bit of the last twenty-four years. (I cannot say the same thing for the first thirty years of my life.) I remember the joy I felt when my daughter and son were born; the sadness and trials as well as the triumphs of their growing up; owning and operating my own business; being a girl and boy scout leader; supporting my daughter's dance lessons and my son's sports and musical instrument classes; etc., etc.

I recall all of it because I am alive by the Grace of God and sobriety...no alcoholic drink or drunk ever gave me any of this.

The glory of sobriety is having the privileged opportunity of enjoying the benefits of being sober.

God bless you all!

Biography

Baptized and confirmed Maria Therese Rosa Catalano. I was born in Hollywood, California, September 28, 1953. Oldest of five children I was raised in the towns of West Covina and Glendora, California, where my parents live today.

I went to college and have a degree in art.

I'm the proud mother of a daughter and son – both outrageously beautiful and handsomely talented.

I am a children's storyteller.

I want to thank Faith for always supporting my children and me the last twenty years.

Discussion/Reflection Questions:

1. What is the payoff for being an addict...a drunk?

2. What is the payoff for being clean and sober?

3. What choices bring you a peaceful, joy-filled heart?

Following Directions

Jane Claypool

Like most drunks, I was driven to sobriety because I needed to stop the pain. I wasn't expecting any payoffs except some relief from the chronic physical and mental illness that I was creating for myself. As we say in the program, "I was sick and tired of being sick and tired."

I wasn't thinking about much of anything when I made the choice to sober up. I didn't really want to reform nor was I ambitious enough to try and bolster my writing career. All my relationships were dreadful but I didn't get sober to please my loved ones. In fact, I needed excuses to support my addictive behavior so I told myself that I drank because they didn't please me!

I wasn't hungry to be a better person. I wasn't worried about my health although I should have been. I wasn't worried about the risks I was taking because I wasn't sure if I cared if I lived or died. Toward the last phase of my active alcoholism, I knew I was suicidal and more than once when I was in a drunken stupor, I left myself a note saying I hoped I would die soon.

The decision to stop drinking was a desperate decision and all I could see was a small dim light in the long, dark, cramped tunnel of my life. I stopped drinking one day when I woke up, looked in the mirror and said to myself, "This is not what I planned to become." It was a first step but it honestly didn't look or feel all that different from many other mornings when I faced the despair of my hangovers.

I think now that my sobriety was a gift from God but I didn't even believe in God at that time and I didn't really understand the gift that morning. I'm still not sure what made the difference between that morning and many others that preceded it. I certainly wasn't optimistic about the future or thinking in terms of gifts from God. All I wanted was to ease the desperate, dark, depressing feelings that came with years of too much booze, too much self-condemnation and too much disappointment with life and myself.

In the beginning, I went to 12 Step meetings because I had seen them work in my two brothers' lives. I'd tried to stop on my own before and failed so I decided to try the meetings. When I got there, people told me to sit down and I sat. Other people told me to listen and I did. Someone gave me a phone number and told me to call her so I did. I was absolutely clueless about what to do next so it seemed like a good idea to follow other people's orders. I was ready to surrender. I knew I needed help and I had just enough sense to know I couldn't trust myself. I was ready to change and I knew that I had to take someone else's advice if I was going to succeed.

While I was never hospitalized or put in jail, I was at the bottom of my barrel and couldn't climb out without help. I was living in Mexico, my money was running out and so were my friends. Most had simply disappeared because I was too hard to be around when I was drinking and I was nearly always drinking. Even though most of the people in my 12 step meetings were Spanish speaking men, I found some Americans and I could speak some Spanish so I heard what I was supposed to hear.

When I tell people that I got sober in Spanish speaking meetings filled with male campesinos, my story surprises them. It is true that I lacked fluency in the language but I could understand the simple directives and sense the atmosphere of comradeship. I found being a foreigner healing in many ways because I was free of the fear of comparisons that haunted me in my home culture. At home I felt like a failure. In Mexico, I was simply Juanita, or at most la professora, and I felt free to change and to be me. It seemed comfortable because no one was judging me.

That was 32 years ago at this writing and, in retrospect, I see that my sobriety really was a gift from God and the person who was judging me was myself. God offered me a gift and I accepted it only because I was thoroughly exhausted by my alcoholism. I wake every morning filled with gratitude for the changes I've found since that wonderful day.

The first changes in my life seemed remarkable. All those changes came about because I listened to "them" and did what I was told. They told me to practice gratitude and I started making a daily list of things I was grateful for. I still do that as a part of my spiritual practice.

They told me to make amends and I really tried. It was hard for me to humble myself and ask for forgiveness but it worked. Within a few months, my relationships were mostly healed. Although I had to give up my drinking buddies and stop letting freeloaders take advantage of my relative prosperity, I attracted wonderful new friends. They told me to make amends and I went to all the people I could find that I'd hurt and told them how sorry I was. A few said they didn't want to be friends anymore but most said they loved me and wanted me to be well. Best of all, the estrangement with my family was healed.

Since I was running out of money, I made the choice to go back to the States and try and find work. It was frightening to look for work at age 43 but I was able to get some substitute teaching jobs and then I began writing for the local newspaper. I wasn't a trained journalist so they loved my feature stories and gave me a job in the office but kept passing me over when reporting jobs were open. It was discouraging but I kept going to meetings and doing my spiritual work. I was grateful to have money for food and rent and trying hard not to resent the fact that the newspaper kept hiring young men just out of college for the jobs I so wanted.

Then another miracle happened! Before I'd gone to Mexico

to live and drink, I'd sold a novel to a large publishing company. They gave me an advance check but never published the book. That became another excuse for drinking and I continued to write but never really got it together to make a true effort in my drinking days. Once I was sober, I was in a position to take care of business and I did. After ten years of writing unsuccessfully, I was able to establish a wonderful writing career within a few months. By the end of my third year of sobriety I was on the New York Times best seller list for teen age fiction. My dreams were coming true and all because I was sober.

The road to writing success was not easy but it was nothing compared to the trouble I'd experienced when I was drinking. In order to make it in the writing world, I had to step out and take risks. I also had to work hard and follow directions. When I was drinking, I wrote every day but I couldn't work very hard and I certainly couldn't follow directions. I learned about the business of publishing. I started following the writer's guidelines for material I submitted to publishers. I also overcame my shyness and feeling of "not being enough" and tried to network with people who could help me. The lifestyle changes I made in sobriety enabled me to succeed in my deepest and most heartfelt desire.

Because I was living on the East Coast, I began to spend time in New York City publisher's offices and I started taking assignments. These assignments meant money in the bank and they also guaranteed that I would be recognized as a writer. They were important to me and I was very eager to succeed. One time, I was quite nervous about an interview with a book editor who I hoped would offer me a book contract.

This opportunity meant a great deal to me and I was literally shaking as I got off the train and started walking toward the publishing company. I was so nervous I thought I needed to go to the toilet before the interview in spite of the fact that I was running late. Although I had been sober for a few years and had achieved a certain amount of success and peace of mind, I believed that this particular contract was the gateway to my future. For some reason, it felt like a make or break appointment and I was scared.

I was so nervous that I thought if I failed to heed the call I might have an accident. I went into a hotel and used the ladies room. Then, on the way out, I popped a button on my suit jacket. The button rolled back into the corner of the toilet stall and I had to get down on my hands and knees to rescue it. Once down on my knees, I looked into the toilet tank and burst out laughing. All I could think about was the many times I'd been in exactly that position so I could throw up after a bout of wine drinking. How could one appointment be as scary as the tight spots I'd been in the past?

Laughter is a great leveler and it helps keep people like me sane. On my knees, I asked myself, "How important is it?" and I realized that I'd better stop scaring myself and live a day at a time as I'd been taught. My nervousness disappeared and I sailed through the interview without a moment's hesitation. I was so grateful for the gift of sobriety that I honestly didn't worry anymore about whether or not I got the contract. I did get the job and many, many more over the next ten years.

My successful writing career is only one of the gifts that sobriety brought me. Those gifts span every area of my life. My personal relationships are all good. My health isn't great at this age but I am still here and considering how I treated my body for years, I am truly grateful for life at age 75. My work life has been a phenomenal success with the writing and then later my choice to become a Religious Science minister. I'm truly amazed at how much more I received from life than I could even have imagined those many years ago.

After building my writing career and enjoying that success, I decided that Spirit was calling me to the ministry and I began to take Science of Mind classes with the intention of becoming a minister. It took me six and a half years to complete all the requirements and then I set out to start my own church. I started a church and it is still in existence. During my career as a minister, I wrote three spiritual books and trained over thirty Religious Science ministers. I also served on the Board of Education and the Board of Directors of Religious Science International. In 2000 I was awarded the Raymond Charles Barker award for writing. I was also awarded an honorary doctorate for my service to the organization.

As I studied for the ministry, I depended greatly on the lessons of my own life and the wonderful philosophy I'd learned in my 12 step meetings. In my opinion, these ideas blend right into Science of Mind. The first of these ideas has to do with service. The second meeting I attended, down in Oaxaca, Mexico so many years ago, I was told to make the coffee. My first reaction was to resist because I felt sick and it seemed to me everyone else was a lot healthier and happier than I was. But I made the coffee and I felt better. Over the years, I learned that being in service to others is the key to a healthy self esteem and to getting what you want in life. When you are in service, you are giving to others and it is perfectly natural that others give to you.

Another important lesson I learned so long ago was to, "Stick with the winners." I was told that I needed to stay away from, people, places and things that could serve as triggers and endanger my sobriety. Many years later, I would be creating Sunday morning lectures on the Law of Attraction and that would be a slightly different way of advising people to stick with the winners. What we think about tends to come about in our lives so it is important to stick with persons, places and things that make us feel good and release the things that trigger our problems.

As a minister, I have worked with many men and women

who have addiction issues and I feel glad that my background helps me to understand them and point them in the direction of success. Of course, every person must travel his or her individual path but it truly helps to know that someone is there and understands you.

Times change but some things remain the same. When I talk with someone who is struggling with alcohol issues, I remember how it was for me and I thank God I can offer hope. In today's world, most people have treatment centers to help them as well as 12 step meetings. That is a good thing. However, most young people compound their alcohol problems with drug issues. They get into trouble at a younger age and with God's help they get back on track sooner.

Most of my ministerial work is with ordinary people with ordinary problems and I share what I have learned the hard way with gratitude and love. One of the greatest payoffs of the ministry has been my work with my Wise Woman groups and events. Over the years I have trained many women to lead Wise Women groups and help women understand their personal power and their great potential. I have also led Wise Ministers retreats for some of my colleagues every year.

Most of all, I love my Wise Woman Weekends that I lead with two friends and colleagues. Once a year, for the past 15 years, we take between 60 and 80 women on retreat in a comfortable desert hotel where there are many spa offerings and nine mineral pools. We do our workshops in the mornings and evenings and give them the afternoons to have fun, relax, process what they are learning or simply take a nap. It is all part of what we are teaching which is to love and honor yourself and your God-given potential. Our workshops are about basic issues such as relationships, sex, time, money, and health. We help women make choices from the standpoint of their power and give up the idea that they are victims. My book, *Wise Women don't worry, Wise Women don't sing the blues* was published in 1994 and is still selling well.

The ministry, my Wise Women work, my spiritual books and just about everything I have done in my life are based on my belief that being in service is the first and most important part of the glories of sobriety. There is nothing better than reaching out in love to share with others. Before sobriety, even if I could have done what I do, I would have done it with a spirit of competition and I probably would have quarreled with anyone who had any authority over me. I would also have quarreled with anyone who wanted to work in committee because when I was drinking, I was desperate to prove that I was all right. I never even think of those things now. I am comfortable in my skin and willing to let others be who they are.

My life as a loving mother, grandmother, sister, aunt and friend are all dependent on what I learned when I was getting sober. My spiritual program as a Religious Science student, teacher and minister is inseparable from my sobriety. Staying sober a day at a time makes me who I am today. I live in the now quite comfortably. Living in the now is an important part of my life. I must release the past and stop worrying about the future in order to enjoy the moments of this day. When I was first sober, I had so much regret and so much guilt about things I had done in the past that I really had to learn to say, "The past is gone forever," and let it go. Now I know that every day is an opportunity to create a new life and that the past never needs to influence or harm us when we can stay in the now.

Living twenty four hours at a time, sticking with the winners, understanding that service is the key to happiness are all important beliefs that I hold today. Those beliefs give me peace of mind, love of myself and other people and confidence that I will succeed. I am so glad that sobriety has brought me so much and I am filled with gratitude. Each morning I wake up, roll over and say to myself, "Another day to be glad in." I wish the same for you, dear reader.

Biography

Dr. Jane Claypool is founding pastor of the Carlsbad, CA Church of Religious Science. She is also author of over 80 books, writing under the names, Jane Claypool, Jane Claypool Miner and Veronica Ladd. Her teenage books have sold over two million copies and been translated into seven languages. She was awarded the 1981 writer of the year from the Society of Children's Book Writers and the Religious Science International Raymond Charles Barker writing award in 2000. For information about Wise Woman events contact her at WiseJaneC@aol.com.

Discussion/Reflection Questions

1. What is the point of making amends?

2. How does gratitude impact your life?

3. How important is it to follow directions?

Working with Others

Debrah Constance
with Dr. Gideon Haimovitz

A quote from my hero Harriet Tubman: "I looked at my hands to see if I was the same person…there was such glory over everything…the sun came up like gold through the trees and I felt like I was in heaven…." This is what sobriety means to me.

Sobriety is the hope of a better future for all of us and it is the idea that one person can make a change. First of all I don't have the answers. I can only give insight based on my successes as a recovering alcoholic and drug addict. Somebody once asked me the question, "What do you want to do with your life?" That seems like such a simple question. A question that should have been asked of me in the seventh grade but instead I was 44 years old and sober. Something changed in me and this question brought about the following in my life:

> Vice President of Jon Douglas Realty
>
> Founder "A Place Called Home" youth center in South Central Los Angeles
>
> 1997 President's Summit for Americas Future Award
>
> 2002 World Sacred Music Festival Award with the Dali Lama
>
> My autobiography *Fat, Stupid and Ugly (One Woman's Courage to Survive)*
>
> A made for TV movie about my life by Lifetime TV network
>
> And much, much more…

This is just a short list of some of my accomplishments and they are a direct result of my sobriety. My life has brought me so much joy, pain and love that I felt the need to share it with those who had just the pain.

One minute I was causing so much damage to all those who loved me and the next I was attempting to repair this damage. It amazed me how easily one can tear apart her life and yet how difficult it is to rebuild it. I think the path to rebuilding determines your success in a twelve step program. I was serious about my rehabilitation in this world and I was ready to start building. This is a look at my rebuilding and how this was the key to my sobriety.

Many imagine alcoholics in some demonic form: people who hate not only themselves, but also everybody around them; people who destroy everything and can't live a normal life. Or, as street people who must not be taking care of their families. In fact these "demons" we see as alcoholics are usually people all around us who we would never guess are struggling so hard every day.

I was an alcoholic who functioned as a normal person and did so diligently my entire life. I was the mother and hard worker who nobody would have guessed had so many demons inside. My demons were very well hidden in order to protect myself and my family. I did not have the tools to survive without drugs and alcohol. My family robbed me of my childhood and also of my ability to survive in this world without numbing myself from the daily realities. My only hope and means of survival at a young age were my friends, and as an adult, was my son Gideon. I had to be there for him and it was the hope that he would have a better life than I had that kept me going.

I did not know I was an alcoholic. The demon just grew inside without my knowledge or awareness and one day I woke up and found myself desperate to make a change. This change was a drug rehab hospital program, my training ground to learn principles of life and how to deal with what my parents never taught me. It was here that I learned to cope with my past and dig into the future with new hope for all the possibilities that life could now offer. I was now able to function in the world. It wasn't that simple; my story is much longer and much more involved. My success as a recovering alcoholic depended on following the 12 Step program that Alcoholics Anonymous outlines and getting a sponsor that would support me in the program. I spent a lot of time in AA, meeting after meeting, and it was here that I learned what can happen when you work with others. I had been a taker and did not realize it. I thought that I was the best mom, wife and employee but the reality was I robbed all of them of me. I was so inebriated all of the time, how could I be there for any of them? Sobriety taught me to forgive myself for my mistakes, to take a new breath of fresh air and to allow myself to be the person that I had always envisioned.

I now had the tools and the answer to the question, "What do I want to do with my life?" This question was important for so many reasons. I wanted to help others and believed that one person helping another could bring about a psychic change in this world. It was time to be honest with myself and even though I never graduated from high school and had lived a tough life, from this moment forward I wanted to be there for others. It gets easier when you surround yourself with the monumental task of being bigger than yourself. What I mean is, finally I could focus on not only healing myself but sharing this bigger knowledge of healing with others.

It was at this point that I started volunteering for different charitable organizations. This led me to the point where I resigned from a six-figure income at Jon Douglas Realty, which at the time was the number one real estate company in greater Los Angeles. It was at this moment that I put my foot forward and started "A Place Called Home" (APCH). APCH was the culmination of really wanting to make a positive change in this world and APCH was the new home for me to share my heart and soul with others that needed it. I was on the path forward, not backward, and always thanking my guardian angels for getting me this far. APCH is a youth center in South Central Los Angeles and is my vision of how the world should be. In APCH there are no colors, races, or sexes...we are all just one family of different skin tones, different religions and different gang territories. Yet we are all one family and I was the mother hen to over 500 young children in the beginning and to over 5000 at my retirement. All the awards and accolades I received were nothing in comparison to helping one child that was in trouble. I liked helping the really troubled children. I could relate so well to the children who were really hurting. In fact I think I attracted them. I was the mother hen and this was a beautiful time when I knew that I was making a difference in this world. I could see the changes in their behavior, the joy in their faces and the laughter in their voices. I wanted to be there for this family and share the love that I always wanted for my own family with this much larger one.

I guess people saw me as a hero but I just think if everyone did one small thing for someone else, this would amount to amazing change in this world. Don't just give someone money; give them a hand. That is what this world needs.

Hope is a chant, a chorus and a dance.

Hope is a child who discovers the magic of books.

Hope is a mentor who opens his life to a teenager from South Central.

Hope is a volunteer who shows up week after week.

Hope is a gangbanger who learns to play guitar.

Hope is a shy and awkward youth who blossoms into a graceful dancer.

Hope helps us see beyond our boundaries.

It helps us wake up each day.

It helps us believe.

It keeps us coming back in the face of frustration and doubt.

It fuels our dreams.

Hope is a universal language.

(The above is an excerpt from *Fat, Stupid and Ugly*)

Hope is our ability to see the silver lining in the clouds and to create a better tomorrow for ourselves and those that we love. Why don't we start spreading some hope in this world and help each other instead of hurting everyone around us? AA saved me and I hope that someone reads this and shares my hope of a better world with others.

Biography

Debrah grew up in New York and Milwaukee, and at age 19 moved to California where she worked for her uncle in his Hollywood advertising agency.

Debrah left advertising and in September 1993 organized and opened the doors of A Place Called Home (APCH). From that first day, when 12 children showed up, to today, where APCH serves hundreds of children and has a membership of nearly four thousand, she has worked tirelessly to help children have safer lives and realize bigger dreams.

Recently, Deborah survived a near-fatal car crash, found the love of her life, and has now scaled back her work at APCH.

Discussion/Reflection Questions

1. How would working with another person assist you in developing viable solutions to your current situation?

2. Please write a "gratitude list" that you can be proud of and consider sharing it with someone else to help him or her get sober.

Reflections of Joy

Rebecca Flood

Sitting here today I realize that I have been granted a spiritual reprieve of 12,130 days from the suffering of my chronic and incurable disease. I am also reminded that in these days I have lived a joyous, happy and free life just by maintaining total abstinence from all mind-altering chemicals. This reprieve has provided opportunities beyond any I could have imagined as one who was addicted to alcohol, pills and pot. A dear friend has a mantra that she shares with newly recovered addicts: "I will stay sober for the rest of my life, one day at a time, no matter what." In truth, that is how I have lived my life, both consciously and subconsciously, for the past 33 years. As a result of this determination and the practice of living a spiritually based life, I have reaped many rewards and experienced many glories. How amazing is that?

The program that I attempt to live on a daily basis has promised me many things. Those promises continue to come true regularly. Some have come more slowly than others just as the Big Book of Alcoholics Anonymous ("Big Book") indicates, but they have all been true at various points in my life. Another thing that the Big Book and the Bible say is "Faith without works is dead." My entire recovery and all of the glories I have experienced are a combination of two things: faith and action. Promises in the Big Book are the result of working an honest life and faithfully practicing the recovery principles. What are these promises?

I have just described how amazing my recovery walk has been. *Being amazed* is the first of the twelve promises.

The second promise is *freedom and happiness*. I have experienced freedom from the physical effects of addiction, and freedom to become the person that my Higher Power, whom I choose to call God, intended me to be. I completed a master's degree – pretty remarkable for a woman who flunked the first and third grades and was diagnosed with dyslexia as a child, long before what we know today about the disorder. Abraham Lincoln once said, "We are as happy as we make up our minds to be." However, when one's mind is clouded by mood altering chemicals, it is difficult to be happy or positive. For more than three decades I have spent most of my time content to live life to the fullest, one day at a time, without dwelling in the past or anticipating the future. The result has been unspeakable freedom and happiness.

My only career goal was to help other addicted individuals experience the joy I found. I have always lived by the code to do my best at whatever task is before me, with faith that whatever is meant to be will be. That is exactly what has happened. I surrendered my life to God, my Higher Power. Walking in faith has allowed me to move from a low entry-level job to being the Chief Executive Officer of a non-profit organization. My entire career has brought much happiness to me and to those that love me.

The third promise is *not regretting your past*. Reflecting over my past, I realize that my past and my future are inextricably linked. I am a product of my past. My experiences, good and bad, have helped shape my present and provide direction for my future. I have no regrets for what I have gone through because I have become a stronger person as a result of my life experiences. It was extremely difficult to experience two miscarriages and one premature stillbirth. It was painful to have delivered my third child prematurely and leave him in the neonatal intensive care unit after my discharge. Yet today, he is a senior in college, graduating 8th in his high school class, with honors, the captain of his basketball team. He is also the father of my youngest granddaughter and a wonderful father he is. He is a gift as are the other three remarkable children I have had the opportunity to raise. Watching them grow, struggle, learn, love, laugh, face their tribulations and reach adulthood has given me no greater joy. My daughter is the mother of four children only one of whom is her biological child. She has raised her husbands' child since birth and has adopted two children who are siblings. She is also a senior in college working on a degree in early childhood education while working full time as the operating room coordinator in her local hospital. What mother would not be proud? Despite many problems with my oldest son as an adolescent, today he is a union electrician happily married to an occupational therapist and expecting his first child. My youngest is still an adolescent and just started his freshman year in high school. He is developing into who he will be and, at the same time is challenging his stepfather and me. He is a gifted writer, basketball player and often wise beyond his 14 years. However, he is still an adolescent and I am hopeful all three of us will survive this period. I do not know how the lives of my children will turn out or what difficulties and challenges they will face. I continue to love and support them, and have faith that I have given them my best. Now as they are adults I can be their friend as well. That too is a joy and a blessing.

So, why should I regret that their father was never committed to family or that I was a single mother for 10 years raising my own children and caring for three God-daughters whose mother was struggling with addiction? Yes, there were hard times. But never did I allow myself the luxury of self-pity or regrets. And today, I am blessed with loving, productive children. Without the unfortunate and painful marriage this would not be the case. Without the loss of a prior marriage I would never have been motivated to enter counseling, which helped me choose new and different relationships.

Today I am happily married to a man I consider my soul mate. My husband is purely a gift of right living and an absolute joy. We have our struggles, differences and difficulties but there is only one option and that is that we are in this together no matter what. With that relationship comes a blended family consisting of 6 children, 5 grand children (so far), 4 dogs, and 2 cats.

The lesson for me is clear: do not spend any emotional energy regretting the past but stay in the present. It is so much more enjoyable and real. Regrets may surface regarding things that happened, things we wish we had done differently. Often, it is not until years later that we can let go of the guilt, shame and remorse those regrets bring. If we keep the faith and hold our heads high, we will often find that the things we regret most bring us the greatest gifts of all.

The fourth promise is that *you will comprehend the word serenity and know peace.* During my years of recovery I have slowly and I mean very slowly begun to understand what true serenity and peace are. I cannot begin to describe how wonderful it is to be able to sit quietly at peace with myself with no noise, other person, or thing to divert my attention from my own thoughts and emotions. It has taken much time and practice and today I yearn for solitude, quiet and time to just be. Practicing the healing arts of meditation, yoga, message, reading, listening to classical music and kneeling in prayer alone in a chapel – feeling God's presence – these activities have helped me to center and find serenity and inner peace.

Alcoholics Anonymous promises that *you will see how your experiences benefit others.* As I have been open to my Higher Power I can see this is true. In my life's work I have developed treatment programs for adolescents afflicted by addiction and most often a mental health diagnosis or learning disability, and designed and implemented treatment services for women who are pregnant or parenting so that their children can remain with them while in treatment. Practicing the Golden Rule to "do unto others as you would have done to you" I am overcome with how many people have made footprints in my life and how many footprints I have made in the lives of others. It can take your breath away.

The next promise is that *uselessness and self-pity will disappear.* I have found that when I am focused on helping others and doing the work that is in front of me there is no time for self-pity. I am too busy to feel useless. This just flowed into the seventh promise: *you will lose interest in selfish things and gain interest in our fellows.* When I accepted who I was (an individual with an incurable addictive disease over which I have no control), surrendered to my Higher Power, began to experience peace within myself, I began to feel a genuine interest in others and less concern for myself. In fact, my interest in helping others became all-consuming and was a major source of my joy. It is difficult to explain. Perhaps it is best expressed in the Bible in Matthew 16:25, which says: "For whoever wants to save his life will lose it, but whoever loses his life for me will find it." This interest and concern for others continues to be the focal point of my life.

A natural result is the eighth promise, which is *self-seeking will slip away.* And that is exactly what happened and it has never returned. Promise number nine was a direct result of the first eight: *your whole attitude and outlook on life will change.* Life to me today is a precious gift. I am primarily an optimistic person who believes in the good of others. I have a desire to be of service wherever I can be. That is a 180-degree turn from abusing my body with chemicals and attempting to feel good by ingesting alcohol, pills and marijuana. Yes, having a new outlook on life is truly one of the glories of sobriety.

The next promise is another tough one for me. It took years for me to realize that my anger toward myself and others was really masking a multitude of fears. Promise number ten is *fear of people and economic insecurity will leave us.* My greatest revelation was realizing what a fearful person I was, both of

47

people and financial security. Alcoholics Anonymous promises that these fears will slip away. And believe it or not I get glimpses of this every day. It is not complete, which means I have more work to do here. I have always been afraid to speak in front of people, worried what people really think of me. As a result of just facing these fears, speaking publicly, accepting myself, getting to know people, taking risks with people, much of this has left me. One of my greatest fears was loosing my Mother. She was the only one who, when I was a rebellious, angry, teenage alcoholic and drug addict, never lost faith in me. She never spoke one negative word. Rather, she loved me unconditionally and was my confidant. There was nothing I could not talk about with my Mother. I became very attached and depended on her when I failed to trust others. While I knew that she would one day pass, I lived in fear of the thought. That day has come and gone. She passed away four years ago. I survived my greatest loss. Some days feel like I am just surviving but when I move beyond the grief and into the joy I experienced just having had such an unbelievably wonderful mother and extraordinary friend, I feel blessed and am filled with gratitude. I was truly blessed to have had her for as long as I did. So sometimes in facing our fears we are given gifts. Again I say action and faith is the key.

A great struggle as a single mother and sole breadwinner was having enough money. For over a decade, in order to pay the bills I worked three jobs: a primary job, a part-time counseling job and a job cleaning offices. Today I am not sure how I did it but back then, you just did it. My children share with me fond memories of those years that I felt were such a struggle. They remember playing hide-n-seek in the offices while I cleaned or watching Disney movies and eating popcorn in one office while I was counseling in another. So even though those were difficult and fearful times they were also filled with joy and love.

I can remember so many times that I did not know how I was going to pay to get my car repaired or pay for the shoes my son needed to play ball, or hoping the $10 for gas would get me to and from work. Instead of staying stuck in the fear I got into action and learned how to budget, how to invest, how to save.

The eleventh promise is one that just happens for me. I am still not always sure how. This promise is: *you will intuitively know how to handle situations that used to baffle you.* As situations present themselves I generally just deal with them. Most times I look back and I am comfortable with the results. Often I am amazed that I handled things so well. People in my professional life frequently tell me how well I get the job done. However, I believe when you leave room for grace and mercy and get out of your own way it gives God room to do the work.

The biggest and most rewarding promise is number twelve: *you will suddenly realize that God is doing for you what you could not do for yourself.* I finally realized that God was present in all aspects of my life and was working on my behalf even when it did not seem like it to me. Believing in God, a power greater than yourself, Jesus, or whatever fits for you, is the greatest and most sustaining gift one can ever have and with that all things are possible. As long as you "do not use alcohol or drugs one day at a time no matter what," do the soul work and keep the faith, in the end it is all glorious.

Biography

Since 2004 Rebecca Flood has been the Executive Director and CEO of New Directions for Women in Costa Mesa, California. This non-profit, residential facility assists women and their families suffering from alcohol and drug dependencies. Becky also provides Morningside Recovery in Newport Beach with administrative leadership – assisting people with co-occurring diagnosis. She earned her Masters degree in Human Services from Lincoln University in Pennsylvania, is a Nationally Certified Drug and Alcohol Counselor (NCAC II), and is a Licensed Certified Alcohol and Drug Counselor (LCADC). Becky lives in Southern California with her husband and soul mate, creating a blended family of six children, five grand children, four dogs and two cats.

Discussion/Reflection Questions

1. Which life experiences helped you become a stronger person?

2. Why is "staying in the present" important?

3. How do you find "serenity and inner peace?"

A Day at a Time

Mary Beth Holtzman

My life really began almost 18 years ago when I entered a rehab (due to a family intervention) and began my sobriety. I was 26 years old and I didn't have a clue as to how to live life. I don't mean that I wasn't showing up for work or paying my bills (I was functioning, mostly), I was still able to do that, but I completely lost myself in every way. Up until I began a sober life, life happened to me, I was a constant victim and I had no knowledge of how to live any differently. I was incapable of taking responsibility for any of my experiences and I had no power in my life.

My first drinking binge was at 13. My drinking was periodic for the first few years, then through high school it escalated. When I started college at 18 I became an almost daily drinker. So, needless to say, my only coping mechanism was my best friend, alcohol. I've heard it said that if you drink as an alcoholic, you stop progressing at the age you began drinking. So, I was stuck with a mental capacity of a 13 year old, very fearful girl. Alcohol got me through every challenge, depression, sadness, success, break-up: everything. I truly believe that alcoholism is of the three-fold nature written about in the Big Book: physical, mental and spiritual. I know from my own experience that I had the physical addiction. Every time I put alcohol into my body it set off a physical craving and I had no control over how much I would drink. The mental obsession was very easy to identify with too, no matter how many times I blacked out, passed out, or hurt myself, family, friends, etc., I continued to think that I could have just ONE drink, that I could be one of those "fortunate" people who could control their drinking. I also relate to the Spiritual part of the disease. In fact, looking back at my youth I was spiritually sick. I had no power in my life whatsoever. I believed that God existed, but God wasn't part of my life. God was totally separate from me. I grew up in a very religious family, but I never felt connected to God or really to anyone.

Getting sober and finding a relationship with a God of my own understanding, changed all that for me. The greatest gift I received in sobriety was the freedom to choose the kind of God I wanted to have a relationship with. This has not only allowed me to be sober, but it has opened every door on my journey since. Taking this step in my early recovery was one of the bravest steps I had taken, ever. It was the first time I let go of pleasing others and what they thought of me and taking this step gave me the courage to venture into all the other areas of my life. My relationship with a God of my own understanding has given me courage to realize my dreams. It has given me permission to answer a new kind of "craving" to follow my own Truth, to take a completely different spiritual path than what I was raised with. Taking action and responsibility for my perception on life, today I know that life happens through me. My life experience is a direct result of my daily perceptions. If I'm having a difficult day, I have to stop and look at what is going on with me. Am I not being honest about something? Am I going to enough meetings? Have I been of service? Am I stuck?

I said a number of years ago that if I had made a list of dreams I would like to see manifest in my sobriety, I would have sold myself short. I immersed myself in Alcoholics Anonymous and I focused on staying sober a day at a time. I had many awakenings about myself and my relationship with life (and still do). The "Program" is meant to heal the 3-fold nature of alcoholism (physical, mental and spiritual) and so I became willing to do whatever it took to recover. I took direction and asked for help and I worked on my inner-self. After completing the 12 steps my life changed dramatically. I was able to trust God and practice my new-found courage to let go of my old life. I let go of relationships that were harmful to me. I interviewed for a better job that paid more, and that forced me to learn and grow in my career. I also started making decisions like an adult woman of my age and stopped living from "where is mine" and "I did all this for you, why aren't you doing what I need/want?" I stopped looking to outside things (relationships, material things, even friendships) to fill up that bottomless spiritual hole I had always had. I found that being of service to others filled me with an abundance of Joy. One of my greatest joys of sobriety is helping others on their spiritual journey, whether it's "carrying the message of sobriety" or just being there listening to someone in need.

As I began to face life with this new-found attitude my outside life began taking off. Having learned so much about myself through this process (I was in a survival way of life before I got sober), I was able to make conscious decisions and choices.

In my fourth year of sobriety I met my husband. He also is sober; in fact we had many of the same friends in those beginning years though he and I didn't meet during that time. We have said that God didn't bring us together until we were "ready" (or spiritually whole). I finally accepted someone as a partner who is kind, considerate and respectful. I had changed and was willing to be treated in this manner and I also treat him in the same manner. If I had met him any sooner it wouldn't have worked. He and I were raised in completely different religions, but we share our spiritual way of life together and that works for us. We found a church that resonates with both of us. Living a sober life and practicing the principles gave me the courage to try something different than what I was raised with. It was very scary at first choosing a different religious/spiritual path, but I realized that this is my life and I needed to be honest and true to myself, to be authentic.

I went back to college, taking many spiritual classes and I also was involved in a small theatre group for a while. These are all things that I would have never had the courage to do, had it not been for my sobriety.

After being married for a few years we began praying to have a child. Before our 4th wedding anniversary we had a beautiful, healthy boy. Almost three years later, we had another beautiful, healthy boy.

Being a parent is so much more amazing than I ever imagined. I can't even articulate the amount of joy two beings have brought to my life. Our boys are my teachers and they are constant reminders of God's Grace in my life. One of my dreams was to be able to stay at home and raise our boys especially while they are young. This dream manifested itself when our first son was 10 months old. It was a leap of faith, especially financially. Our financial picture continued to grow in prosperity and abundance. Together we started a small company and after our 2nd son was born, my husband focused on the business and I focused on our family. We continued to prosper in business and at home.

Another Joy of life that I have given myself is to start singing. I always loved to sing, but never took it very seriously. I grew up playing many instruments and being in musicals, etc. I began this journey very simply by joining our church choir and I've been singing in it for many years. I decided to try private voice lessons and I've learned so much about the process I now sing with 2 other friends; we have a singing trio and we have been singing, recording and performing together for over 2 years. Again, this is a direct result of staying sober, taking chances, and being open to my greater good – a day a time.

Recently, I've had some challenges too; it's just "life on life's terms." I have been overwhelmed with experiencing a challenging time, financially. We basically lost most of our material possessions and the business we built is gone. My husband and I both feel that this experience has really shown us that God is our source. God showed up in so many ways to help us through these times. Our wonderful and loving families and friends have been there for us.

I am so grateful to be sober and present during this time and every day of my life. I have been blessed with so many gifts: loving relationships with my husband and children, my family, in-laws and friends, and the ability to create through music or however else I choose. I realize that it's not the big milestones that make a life; it's the day-to-day little things that make up my life and build my future. It is so important for my soul to experience joy no matter what I am going through. How do I choose to be today? I choose to be joyful!!

Biography

Mary Beth began her sobriety in 1990. She grew up in central New York State and has lived in southern California for the last 20 years. Her husband, Stuart, and their boys, Joshua and Sammy, currently live in south Orange County and enjoy the sunshine, the beauty and their wonderful family and friends. Together, she and Stuart founded a non-profit called "Sharing Wellness," which pays for holistic treatments that aren't typically covered by insurance, providing for patients who aren't able to afford such treatments. She actively participates in 12 step programs to continue her sobriety and further her spiritual life. Mary Beth and her family are members of The Capistrano Valley Center for Spiritual Living and she is a Licensed Prayer Practitioner, a teacher in the youth church, and a member of the choir. She also sings with the Shades of Light trio, providing beautiful music and harmonies. Mary Beth continues on her quest for spiritual truths through classes and retreats. As her children are of school age now, she looks forward to this next part of her journey and all the infinite possibilities for creating a joyous, sober life!

Discussion/Reflection Questions

1. Am I taking good care of myself – spiritually, mentally, and physically?

2. Do I have a consistent, daily, spiritual practice – such as prayer, meditation, or journaling – to connect with my Higher Power and be present in the moment?

3. How can I bring joy into my everyday life?

Drunk with the Wine of Life

Maureen Hoyt

The wedding was on the beach about 25 yards from the shore. Bobby, the groom, was sporting toenails painted a bright candy-apple red. It was his way of honoring his younger brother, Robert, who'd passed away unexpectedly three years earlier. When the three brothers were younger, Robert used to get up in the middle of the night and paint their toenails. Being young and not that observant, his brothers would go off to school in their flip-flops, not noticing their painted nails, and Robert would crack up when they were teased unmercifully as only a sibling can do. The backdrop to the wedding ceremony was an oilrig in the Santa Barbara Channel where Robert had been washed overboard and lost his life.

As we stood under the canopy awaiting the bride as she walked across the sand, Bobby said, "I'm going to throw up." "No, you're not," I said; "These people have come to celebrate your wedding day, and you will not mess it up by barfing in front of them." The ceremony went off without incidence, and in fact, it was poignantly beautiful.

When I do a wedding, I usually show up 45 minutes to an hour before the ceremony so that the bride and groom don't have the added anxiety of wondering where the minister is. This particular day, the invitation had asked the attendees to be there by 4:15 p.m. with the idea that when the actual ceremony took place at five, everyone would be in their places with bright shiny faces. Arriving early, most people had about 75 minutes to sit around and drink before the trolley came to take the guests down to the beach. Many people became significantly inebriated, including the wedding party; hence, the groom's worry about throwing up.

After over 35 years of being drug free and over 19 years of being alcohol free, I know that when we clean up our own consciousness, we cannot continue to have anything less in our circle of influence. Something in me that day decided that I no longer wished to associate with the drinking class. There were so many events in my life of which I have little or no recollection because of my flagrant abuse of alcohol or speed; I could not be even remotely close to being in the moment. Noticing the groom's toenails would not have been possible and the poignancy of the oilrig as the backdrop to the wedding ceremony would have been lost.

As a clean and sober person, my appreciation of the little things is huge. There had been many days that I couldn't rouse myself out of bed, and I lost more than one or two days a month to debilitating migraine headaches from alcohol abuse. I often had difficulty managing even the most mundane tasks. Planning for the future was not an option in those days – all efforts were focused on just getting through the day.

Today, I am drunk with the wine of life. Waking up to the expectancy of a day filled with the subtleties of life is infinitely preferable to waking up on the cold, hard bathroom floor, dazed and unable to cope with any thought of what I might be doing today, much less what I would be doing tomorrow or the next day.

Today, I have a fresh vision for my life on a daily basis. The future holds the promise of happiness, and it is such a hopeful thing. In the movie, *The Bucket List*, the characters played by Morgan Freeman and Jack Nicholson know they are dying, and they create a list of things they want to do before they die. At one point in the movie, they are sitting atop a pyramid looking out over the desert expanse. Morgan's character tells Jack that the Egyptians have a beautiful belief that if you can answer the following two questions in the affirmative, you have lived a full life. The first is: have you found joy in your life? The second is: has your life brought joy to others?

Sobriety has brought joy to my life in so many different ways. It allows me to be fully present when I am with my granddaughter. When you are four years old, there is no past or future; there is only the present moment. There are times when I am preoccupied and my attention is elsewhere. My granddaughter will bring me back with such clarity of purpose by emphatically telling me, "Momo, pay attention," and I can.

Ralph Waldo Emerson said, "For every minute of anger, we lose 60 seconds of happiness." And I say, for every moment of sobriety, I have gained a lifetime of happiness. There were many lost minutes, days, and weeks in my past – but I can create a new future. My teacher, Ernest Holmes, said, "The starting point to creating a better future is deliberately to free our minds of the mistakes of yesterday and feel that they are no longer held against us; they no longer need to be a liability." The starting point for every day is gratitude that I have been given another reprieve, letting go of the mistakes of yesterday and providing me with an opportunity to live life more abundantly. There are many things I want to experience, and my "bucket list" gets longer and longer.

Recently, I attended a workshop where the facilitator told the story of two fishermen – one old and one young – sharing the same stream. The young man was not having any luck at all. The old man was catching fish after fish; however, each time, he'd take out a ruler and measure the fish, and then, he'd unhook the fish and throw it back. After watching this behavior several times, the young man approached him and asked what he was doing and why he was throwing so many fish back. The old man said he was measuring the fish to see if they would fit into his cooking pan at home. For many years before sobriety, the Universe was tossing me fish after fish, which I measured by limited thinking, and I tossed them back because they didn't meet the standards of what I knew then.

Those days were filled with pain. As a spiritually mature, clean and sober person, my life is now predicated on the design of my clear and present vision. There is something within me that is transcendent to what I am experiencing, and there is an awareness of the presence of a greater idea at work in my life. When something goes awry in my life as it often does, my thoughts do not go first to the reactive part of me. Instead, I stop, look, and listen to the Spirit within and become the observer of what is going on.

While I once chose unhappiness over uncertainty, blaming everything and everyone for my problems, especially my unskilled mother, today I take personal responsibility for my own experience.

Living in the present moment, it's all right not to know how it's all going to turn out. The conditions and circumstances of my life are not manipulated by some mysterious and predatory force, as I used to believe. The voice of fear is no longer the controlling influence. I am the "master of my fate and the captain of my soul." What I believe about the conditions and circumstances are what causes me pain. I am a woman of power; I am a woman of authority.

My family doesn't really remember the old me, but suffice it to say, everyone in my circle of influence, including my children and siblings, are all better because I am better. And God willing, one day at a time, this is my life, and I am loving it.

Biography

Maureen Hoyt is a Canadian by birth and a naturalized U.S. citizen. She has two children: Heather, 31 years old, married to Bob Phillips, and Nathan, 26 years old. Her granddaughter, Sydney, is the child of Heather and Bob. Maureen recently celebrated her 13th year as pastor of the Granada Hills Church of Religious Science and her 15th year as a minister. She is an active member of the Department of Children and Family Services and her church has adopted a social worker with nine families in her charge. She is currently working on her first book and prior to becoming a minister worked in the insurance and financial planning fields.

Discussion/Reflection Questions

1. How does sobriety enable you to be "fully present?"

2. What do you think it means to "take personal responsibility for your own experience?"

3. Who is "the master of your fate?"

Freedom to be Me

Brenda Ives

When Faith Strong asked me to write about the Glories of Sobriety, I was overwhelmed and honored. I think about my life, of how very blessed I am just to be alive, let alone to live a life that is filled with an overwhelming amount of blessings, love and laughter.

I shudder at the thought of how my life would have turned out (if I were still alive) if I continued living an alcohol and drug induced life.

Yes, my life is absolutely far beyond anything I could ever have imagined or dreamed it would be. I am overwhelmed with gratitude for all of the blessings I have received in the last twelve years. I am comfortable in my own skin; I am in good physical shape and great health.

I have been happily married for six years, I have a rewarding career that pays me well, and I have emotional stability. I learned that I could be happy regardless of the circumstances. I thoroughly enjoy being a Mom; I do charity work that I love. I really love the spiritual energy that comes from good clean living.

In May 2007, I flew from Southern California to Boulder, Colorado to watch both of my daughters graduate from Colorado University. My 24-year-old daughter, Sierra, graduated with a degree in Economics and my youngest daughter, Shay, graduated with a degree in Environmental Planning and Design. The emotions of gratitude and love were so intense that I felt as though my skin would burst open. My cheeks were cramped from smiling. I sat next to my wonderful husband, my brother "Jerry", and nephew "Collier" at the graduation ceremony. There was a day in my life when no one wanted to spend time with me, let alone for a four-hour ceremony in 100-degree heat in Boulder, Colorado. I was wearing a white pantsuit. I had sweat dripping down my back. However, nothing seemed to faze me except the overwhelming gratitude I felt inside.

Not in my wildest dreams had I imagined watching my daughters graduating from college, and with honors. I stopped drinking and using when my daughters were eleven and thirteen. The feeling I had watching them walk across the stage is difficult to express. I never knew living right would result in such an overwhelming feeling of joy and happiness.

I had created a very complicated life for myself, my daughters and all those that were close to me.

My daughters have different fathers. I was married to Sierra's father for only a few years.

Then I met my youngest daughter's father who was kind, compassionate and caring. My first thought was if he only knew who I really was, so ugly, he would leave. But I ran first, and with his daughter; sigh. I had no self worth and thought I was not worthy of anybody's love including my own.

Before I found Alcoholics Anonymous I was a human fear ball. Every thought and action came from fear. Needless to say, I ran before anyone could run from me. Emotionally unhealthy, I never let anybody inside.

Twelve years ago, when I did not want to admit to having a drug and alcohol problem, my spiritual advisor Junie H. asked me to read the promises. I thought, okay, maybe I'll give this a try... but what is in it for me?

I read the promises before working my 5th step of the 12 Step Program. All of the promises came true, all of them. One day at a time, one minute at a time.

I am grateful that God removed my anger. I was angry at the world, and blamed everyone for my misfortunes; I was angry and violent.

My misfortunes were a result of my drinking: the lying, cheating, denial, the family and friends that I was hurting.

I always felt as though my intentions were so good... then I realized that the road to hell is paved with good intentions. My sobriety has been about actions not intentions. Junie H. always tells me "you get what you get when you do what you do."

This statement is so very true, however, when I was drinking I sure didn't get it. Living the twelve steps of Alcoholics Anonymous has changed my life.

When I first got sober I only saw dark, black and ugly. As I attended Alcoholics Anonymous meetings, slowly I started seeing a light. At first it was a small ray of light, then larger and larger.

I attend Alcoholics Anonymous meetings on a regular basis. I hear that I really do have self worth and that I can hold my head up high with the grace of a woman.

I am overwhelmed at the difference in my life. Today, I am able to look in the mirror and see myself. I am able to be accountable and responsible for my own actions.

I continue to check my motives making sure that they are clear of selfishness and dishonesty. I strive to live a life that includes doing nothing shameful, as I never want to jeopardize the self-esteem I have today. The self-love I have acquired over the years is priceless and worth everything in the world to me.

When I was sober for one year, I remember driving home from work and seeing a sunset for the first time. We have all seen sunsets; I had seen many sunsets. However, I was seeing a sunset and feeling a sunset for the first time. The colors were bright and a feeling of Euphoria came over me. God was right there, in the sunset, in me and everywhere.

Last year I took a trip to Mammoth Mountain. The mountains are beautiful, God's art. I skied and snowboarded with my daughters for the first time in 13 years.

As I was riding up on the chair lift with my daughter and her friend, I was overwhelmed with a feeling of gratitude. The gratitude I feel being clean and sober is a feeling that was non-existent during my drinking days/years. Further, I skied with my best friend that I met when I was four years old. What an incredible gift is sobriety!

My daughters and I go on hikes, ride bikes to the beach, run, shop and play sports together. This is something that I never thought would happen in my life. With the grace of God, my daughters have forgiven me for the years of my drinking.

I enjoy visiting my daughters and know that they don't need to be embarrassed to have me around. My daughters are very proud of their Mom's sobriety. They have many friends that have parents that are practicing alcoholics. Their friends pray, wish, dream of their parents getting sober. Yes, my daughters are proud of me.

Waking up on Saturday and Sunday mornings is fun. I never knew that I could actually enjoy the weekend. I spent so much time recovering from binges and then planning on how I was going to binge again. Looking back it was all just stupid. Stupid is the fact that I thought I was having fun at the time!

I am able to deal with any problems I create, however, since I have been clean and sober my life is pretty darn smooth.

After two years of sobriety and working with an amazing sponsor I asked her how I could ever return the favor of her saving my life and the lives of my children, giving me a second chance at life. My sponsor said that I could repay her by doing for others what she had done with me. I felt eternally grateful for someone teaching me how to be honest, have a family, live without doing shameful things that made me lose sight of any self worth I might have had.

My sponsor will not take credit for any help she has given me. She says the credit goes to God. She told me that I could re-pay her by sponsoring girls just like she did with me.

I thoroughly enjoy sponsoring. It is beautiful to watch my sponsorees acquire smiles from the inside out.

I got married six years ago. I am happily married to a wonderful man who has been with me for 19 years. Oh, needless to say, we have had our problems, since when we met I was drinking a lot, not a good Mom, not a good girlfriend and especially not good to myself.

Today, I have a great relationship with my daughters, my family and my husband. I feel as though my relationships include mutual respect. The simple things in life become HUGE overwhelming gifts of joy.

I have a wonderful career. I have purpose and I enjoy each and every moment of my new life.

One of the greatest gifts of my sobriety is the group of girl-friends that I have acquired. These lady friends are my spiritual family on earth. The spirit, smiles, laughter and love we have is awesome.

And one of my best friends is my daughter's father's wife.

I do not have any secrets and the freedom is hard to put into words: nothing to hide, everything to be grateful for.

Dear God, Thank you for taking care of my daughters.

Dear God, thank you for taking care of me.

Biography

"Dear God, Please take care of my daughters." This is how I started every journal entry during my drinking days.

My name is Brenda Ives. I am a 49-year-old happily married lady. I love calling myself a lady today. I am the proud Mother of two amazingly beautiful young ladies. My sobriety date is June 1, 1996. I have been clean and sober for 12 years, one day at a time, sometimes one minute at a time and by the grace of God.

Discussion/Reflection Questions

1. What does it mean to check your motives before your actions?

2. What are three things the writer sees as the glories of sobriety?

3. What are the symptoms of alcoholic behavior?

Sobriety as a Path Back to Myself

West Leffingwell

Hi, my name is West Leffingwell, I am an alcoholic from Leucadia, California. Sound familiar? I hope for your sake that it does.

Have you ever met anyone who said to another or themselves: "Today I'm going to become an alcoholic." I cannot recall such a person nor did I say that before I experienced the effects of ethyl alcohol. I didn't realize that I was on my way to alcoholism before I was born. Science has shown that alcoholism is a genetic disease not a character fault. The first sign that danger lurked was a craving for sweet foods and sugar. At the time, no one related that ethyl alcohol is simply highoctane sugar. Humans have known for a very long time that alcohol is a byproduct of fermented sugar. Fermentation is the process of microbes and yeasts eating sugar to exist and duplicate. One of the waste products they excrete is ethyl alcohol. That's right, booze is bug poop! Yet, even the brightest of those who use or abuse alcohol, seldom reflect on its origins. So what's the big deal about sugar? I like to ask folks "what's the most important substance you derive from the food you consume?" If you answer anything but blood sugar you would be incorrect. Blood sugar is the fuel that runs our bodies. No physical, mental, or emotional activity takes place without it. Only spiritual activity is sugar free and if we were only spirit sugar would not matter. In addition, the pancreatic imbalances are related emotionally to low self esteem, a "cup 'O courage anyone?"

What does this mean? Are we all doomed to be drunks and substance abusers? Hardly, but it is necessary however to be informed. It is necessary to seek information and assume responsibility for your own life and the quality of life you are willing to create. Life is a participation sport. Being good at a sport requires effort, lots of effort if one is of average capabilities as most of us are.

I made the statement that alcoholism is a genetic disorder or disease. It is critical to understand that all who have the genetic liability do not inherit this disease in the same amounts. On a scale of one to ten, how much did you get? It is vital to understand that one exposure to alcohol, tobacco, narcotics, et al. will activate this disease. Are you ready for this? Even behaviors such as gambling, risk taking and sex can activate the disorder. This is absolutely horrific information! The long and the short of it is painfully complex and simple at the same time. If you inherit at a one level, you could quite possibly use substances and control that use. If you inherit at a ten level abuse control is very rare. The best course of action here is: if you don't start the war in the first place you won't have to finish it. Nice words, but totally unrealistic. Exposure to substances in today's world is virtually inevitable whether they be prescription or "recreational". Becoming "hooked" is most often so subtle that it is not recognized for what it is. Why is that? (I thought you'd never ask). If you have inherited the disorder to a five level and above, when the substance enters your body, your body surrenders control and you, as a person, are dismissed and you become the chemical. It takes over and now directs behavior. These figures are used for purposes of demonstration, personal experiences vary. As defined by Bill's Big Book, *"The demand to repeat a performance of perceived pleasure regardless of consequence,"* hence the term "pleasure disorder". More exactly, when we perceive pleasure a center in our brain sends out chemicals (neurotransmitters) to other brain centers and a program of "sure, I'll have another" is initiated. The term, *altered thinking,* describes this behavior. Most all of us have witnessed an individual change personality after consuming a drink or two. Even closer to home, those of us willing to admit our alcoholism, have no doubt been told by our loved ones that "you were out of control again last night; next time you're walking home". Doing a substance daily is a red flag. Feeling you deserve it is a garrison sized red flag.

In my humble opinion, the primary motivation for using a substance is to change the way I feel. The way I feel is a function of how I perceive the world around me. The way I perceive is based on my belief system(s). Many believe that the human belief system is largely established by three years of age.

The scenario I would like to propose here goes like this: Here you are in the dimension of spirit: you stand in line to sign up for a human experience. You have a definite purpose, a time frame, a location, and have selected the genetics to best aid you in effecting that purpose. You have in your memory system all that has ever been for you. So here we go, BAM, conception occurs and a massive slowdown from spiritual vibratory levels to earth plane is in effect. This is not reassuring. It becomes instantly apparent that it is vital to develop a game plan for survival. And so it begins, there is often a conflict between what we feel and perceive with what in fact is going on. But wait, I'm just a developing entity here, I'm dependent on this mother for my life, and I'm hooked into her food supply, and feelings, and all of her bodily functions good or not so good. The first point here is that right off the starting line we have very little control over those situations around us, yet we must somehow cope with them to survive.

The second point is that the survival strategy that we develop is based on feelings derived from our environment and the events occurring each nanosecond in that environment. A third factor is we seem to be commissioned to forget our memory of past experience (on a conscious level) so that we can have a truly human experience, learning, adapting and creating harmony in our lives through acceptance. Observation seems to indicate that our logic develops more in the seven year age bracket. This would imply that most of our beliefs are formed of emotional perception from conception into the three to five year time frame. It is not a stretch for me to understand that many of these early formed beliefs are based in fear. If much of what goes on in the world scares me, why wouldn't I want to change the way I feel. Now I have another reason to use substances.

You might see by now I'm amassing logic so that changing the way I feel is perfectly OK. This is *altered thinking*. But wait, there's more. The newborn has many of the patterns of life already memorized and imprinted – language, pattern sounds, musical patterns, voice quality – and associated feelings. When we enter the world we are completely at the mercy of the people and environment in which we find ourselves. We aren't mobile, cannot feed ourselves, and cannot care for even our most basic survival needs. Scary? It can be and most likely is at times even in the best of situations.

The embellishment of our belief system continues as our experiences expand. Right at the top of the list of influences is parental behavior. If these people were grand enough to have you as their issue, they must be wonderful. Even though their behavior may be totally dysfunctional and scare the living daylights out of you, it must somehow be of value. The same applies to the environment in which you are developing. Even if you intuitively know that what is going on around you is morally corrupt, there is a high probability you will mimic the behavior.

The perception is that they are surviving doing that so I will survive if I copy. A couple of personal examples: I adopted my mother's belief that there would never be enough money and that violence was a part of being angry. I assumed that when men had spare time after work, at parties, on weekends that the consumption of alcohol and cigarette smoking was what men did. My father was not an angry drunk, he always worked and provided, was quite moral, and was highly respected in the community. So what's not to mimic?

I began smoking cigarettes habitually at age 14 and alcohol occasionally by age 16. I would no doubt have consumed alcohol more often if it was easier to obtain. Thus my journey into substance abuse began. As science has shown, alcohol, nicotine, narcotics, and even behaviors are dose dependent: it takes ever more to get to "normal".

I had the advantage of growing up in a relatively rural environment in Southern California with a few years in Oregon. My parents didn't divorce, I was curious and precocious, and as naïve as any teen. I graduated from the local high school, tried UCLA as an engineering major, worked, saw the light, went back to school, got married, had three children and 6 years later had a D.D.S. after my name. In 1960 I began practicing locally and things prospered.

Five years later things didn't look so rosy. Alcohol had been allowed to destroy much of our lives. By this time there were four children, my wife was a suicidal pill consuming alcoholic who was often institutionalized. I was basically a single parent with an active business and I was using. There was no such thing as insurance for this type of calamity. I was in serious financial trouble paying hospital bills. In retrospect I am amazed that alcohol's grip had blocked my ability to see the cause of my self-induced woes. I filed for divorce and won custody of my children. This occurred in 1965. In those times a husband just did not get custody, meaning that the mother was too far gone to cause any argument. As the children did their best to survive their family life, there were two more marriages before I met my present (and last) wife.

I have always been very fortunate that in my darkest hour, someone sheds light on an optional path. It was through healing my business that I was opened to healing my life. What began with business led me to quit alcohol and anything else I used. This event occurred on June 24, 1984 at

6:30 PM, my mother's birthday. I ordered a whiskey sour, had a sip, almost hurled it, and that was the end of it. No more, period. I did this cold turkey without a sponsor. I did use the 12 Step approach, I did twelve years of counseling, I attended AA meetings, and I accept the fact that I cannot ever consume alcohol or narcotics. My greatest asset is a loving and supportive wife of twenty-seven years. As it is with all valuable assets, nurturing and respect are mandatory. It is simply too much work to quit again. Stopping the substances is the easy part. Healing the feelings is the arduous part.

Once I had become devoted and committed to staying sober I often found my thoughts reviewing past "mistakes." This regretful reviewing has limited value. Yes, those were really awful things I did while under the influence. No, there will be no more of that because I am and will remain sober and be in present time. I prefer to reflect on all of the truly wonderful things I accomplished during the times I was using. I cannot retrieve any of those events, nor can I change their outcomes. I choose to focus and capitalize on the positives because I like the feeling it gives me in my heart.

The continuance of my healing journey has been greatly enhanced by over thirty years of study in metaphysics and twenty-four years clean and sober. These have aided me in developing an understanding and relationship with the spiritual aspects of our universe. This empowerment enabled me to gain the financial stability and freedom to retire at age 67. I continually endeavor to heal family relationships and I seek sober friends that do not live in the past. I strive to be in and fully enjoy the moment even though the plans may change, to be an expression of my beliefs, to actualize that I am loved, to live in love and gratitude, and to act for my highest and best good.

Surely if I do those things for myself it will be a benefit for you as well. I adamantly surrender all motivations to puff, trip, sip, drop, toot, or shoot. I am completely able to accept and take responsibility for all of my feelings positive or negative. It's not what is going on that matters it's how I deal with it that matters. I am just fine, warts and all!

Biography

Nee: November 23, 1934 La Jolla, California

Education: San Dieguito High, UCLA, Santa Monica City College, Dental Degree: Thomas W. Evans Dental Museum and Institute, Philadelphia, Pennsylvania, 1960.

Retired: 2003

Hobbies: Auto restoration, Metaphysics, Health Consultant, Writing, Cooking, Gardening, Painting, Learning, General Handyman

Discussion/Reflection Questions

1. Your life is an expression of your moment-to-moment choices. What choices do you make daily or even hourly to assist yourself in remaining sober?

2. Besides yourself, who is your greatest human asset? What are you doing to nurture and strengthen that relationship?

3. Assuming you are composed of three parts: a spiritual, a mental/emotional, and a physical, what are you doing to promote sobriety in each of these areas?

Old Enough

Devon Martin

Am I really old enough to be an alcoholic?

I was seventeen when I was introduced to recovery. It was one week before my eighteenth birthday. As a young person, I had not lost all of the *outside* things you hear about – job, house, family, etc. – but drinking and using had taken over my life. I had lost everything – inside. I was told I had to start to identify my feelings. It was very difficult for I had never really talked about how I felt. In the beginning of my sobriety I heard all of the differences: no jail, no kids, no car, and no house. Then at one meeting I heard a woman speaker who said that alcoholic women are ashamed of what they had become. I could really relate to that. I came into the rooms of the Twelve Step Program with so much shame. It was painful just to function throughout the day.

"Just change everything", they said. I was so broken inside I was willing to try anything. *Willing – that is a powerful word.* This was the first time I had ever practiced the concept. I had to be willing to listen, willing to get into action, willing to not think too much, and willing to try to keep my mouth shut. I was told to stop hanging out with my drinking friends – they still made it look good – but if I stopped hanging out with them what would I do for fun? How could I possibly have fun without a keg and my friends? It got so painful and lonely that I started reaching out to some young people at my meetings. It was really awkward. I was not very good in a social situation without my alcohol and drugs. I was asked to go to a sober Twelve Step dance. I did, and liked it. I started going out on a regular basis with my new friends in the Twelve Step Program. I realized I was having fun sober. It was so exciting to go somewhere at night and wake up in the morning and remembering everything.

I was told to get a sponsor. I picked a wonderful woman who scared me. I did everything she told me. I followed her to meetings and started working the steps. I felt that when I did the fourth and fifth step with her, I planted both feet in the Twelve Step Program. She told me that I had a clean slate to start my life over. WOW. Where else could I admit my dark secrets, actions and thoughts, and be told that I could start over? I burned that first fourth step in a fire pit at the beach, and felt I buried my old self as the ashes floated up in the sky.

Sobriety has given me freedom, something that I did not have in my life while drinking and using. For instance, I had the clarity to actually make a decision on my own. I decided to go back to school. Because of my using, I had to redeem myself and my grades before any four-year college would look at me. So I went to a junior college and began the process of asking myself, what do I want to be when I grow up? I had learned in the Twelve Step Program to ask for help, which I had NEVER done; so I went to a college counselor and decided, after much thinking, praying and talking, that I wanted to be an artist. I was encouraged in the Twelve Step Program to follow my dreams. I decided I wanted to go to a small Art College in Pasadena, California; however, I had no idea what to do in order to accomplish this. I was taught that if I took some action, stayed sober, and turned to God, that I could do anything. I submitted the required 12 drawings with high hopes. It took three applications to finally get accepted. I learned much in that process, especially not to give up. When I received the first rejection letter, I wanted to quit trying. Instead, I talked to my sponsor and prayed, and was reminded that this was all in God's time. If I truly wanted this, I needed to keep trudging forward. I shared my feelings about my disappointments, my discouragement and my fears that maybe this was not meant to be. I was constantly reassured and told to keep taking the next step. I finally received an acceptance letter and I was off to pursue a dream – another first for me. I moved to Pasadena, away from the Twelve Step Program that I had known and at which I felt so comfortable for the past 5 years. I was fearful but at the same time excited. I was advised to go to Twelve Step Program meetings immediately when I got to my new city and to be consistent about the meetings I went to so people would get to know me. So I did. I got a coffee commitment and started meeting new people. It was hard, but I knew I HAD to do it to maintain my sobriety, and to not isolate myself – another one of those actions I did not want to take. After some time, I established another strong support group to help me through life, sober.

Through the process of finishing college and becoming an artist I learned not to give up on a dream, to talk about what was really going on in my head, and to trust in people who had more sobriety and experience than I, and to keep taking ACTION. If I had followed my own way I would have never even touched my dream; I would have quit before the miracle happened. For me, if I don't talk about the big and little daily experiences of my life, I'm not sure I would still be enthusiastic about my sobriety and life. In taking productive instead of destructive actions, I started to develop good morals and values and regained some self esteem. My actions resulted in higher self esteem. I always thought I needed to feel my way into better esteem, not act my way into it.

I finished college sober and sane and then had to decide on my career. I know that God had taken me this far, and He was with me, encouraging me to even go further. So, I moved again – to San Francisco – away from my then familiar and supportive Twelve Step Program. I immediately went to a meeting. At that time I had about nine years of sobriety and had come to understand, and really believe, that I could do anything and go anywhere with the help of the Twelve Step

Program and the hand of God. I don't ever have to be alone again. Loneliness was now a choice, not a way of life. When I began going to regular meetings in San Francisco, I made friends immediately. (My roommate, who was not an alcoholic, had a really hard time meeting people.) I got a sponsor, good friends and was a part of life in San Francisco. For me, feeling part of is very important to my sobriety. I am accountable and therefore cherish my sobriety and my life. If I am to stay sober I have to keep my commitment of working the twelve steps and traditions of the Twelve Step Program in my life, being honest with at least one other sober alcoholic woman and attending meetings often.

My career was going well; sobriety was going well; now I started to date. I was told early on in recovery not to get romantically involved with anyone in my first year of sobriety. I followed this suggestion so I could work on myself; I had a lot of cleaning up to do before I could contribute anything to a relationship. Spending that first year without the distraction of dating solidified my place in the Twelve Step Program. I felt comfortable in my own skin due to working the steps, which in turn gave me a new attitude. I knew what I wanted, and would not settle anymore.

After living about a year in San Francisco, I met my husband at a Twelve Step Program meeting. We dated, and then got engaged. We have been married 12 years and have three children. We support each other in our sobriety and walk the same spiritual path. One of my greatest memories from our wedding day was walking down the isle on my Dad's arm. This was a man that I really did not like when I was drinking. I had made amends to him when I had about a year of sobriety. I told him plain and simple how very sorry I was for causing him any pain. That simple amend slowly opened the door to healing. I felt so right with the world and my fellows, and to see all these faces smiling at me, was freeing. These were faces that I had given to and not taken away from or harmed in many years, thanks to my working the Twelve Step Program. Faces, that truly loved me, and I them. I will never forget that moment and am so grateful that God let me experience that day. I felt that the years of being consistent, honest and sober were real when I looked into all those faces. I choose every day to be sober and am thankful that God has given me this gift of sobriety.

Being a mom is a special thing, but being able to be a sober mom is tremendous. I know every time I choose sobriety, I am giving my kids a gift. I can be present for them, and love them unconditionally. When I was drinking and using, I came first no matter what. I struggle daily to be a good mom, a mom that can hold my head up high knowing that I am exactly were God wants me to be. I sometimes grapple with negative thoughts, but I realize now that just because I feel something does not mean that it is true. That is such a freedom.

For the past 24 years of sobriety, I have learned and experienced many things. Feeling doesn't paralyze me anymore. I have the daily gift of freedom to choose. I have choices instead of barriers. I am able to lay my head down on my pillow at night and know that I am all right with God and my fellows. I can ask for help, and take direction. I have tools today to live life – the telephone, praying, writing, helping others, etc. I wake up looking forward to the day instead of dreading it, remembering what I have done and said the prior day. I try to treat people the way I would want to be treated. All of these things I learned in the Twelve Step Program have allowed me to live life the way I feel God really intended me to live.

Often people ask me why I still go to meetings. The truth is, if I don't I start to forget. I start looking from the outside in, instead of the inside out. I become irritable, wanting instead of giving, thinking about myself way too much, not feeling a part of. So I go to meetings to remember – not to feel alone and different.

I hope that the people who know me or meet me see a good example of a sober woman. I have grown up with some incredible men and women who have taught me how to be a woman of integrity. They taught me not to take my sobriety for granted – to respect my disease – to honor the Twelve Step Program. I try to be genuine and loving. I was so blessed to have gotten sober when I did, in Laguna Beach, to have the big arms of the Twelve Step Program wrap around me. I still am very active in the Twelve Step Program and am honored to sponsor other women, helping others chip away at that selfish armor I still try on.

Getting sober at a young age and admitting that I was an alcoholic was not my goal in life. But in doing so, I found joy, a sense of peace and the answer to my question – yes, I WAS old enough.

Biography

I was born in Newport Beach, California in 1966. I grew up in Newport Beach until the age of twelve when we moved to Laguna Beach. I graduated from Laguna Beach High School in 1984. That summer I got sober.

I have been married twelve years and we have three children under the age of ten.

I go to meetings in Newport Beach where I now live.

Discussion/Reflection Questions

1. How can I be an alcoholic, when I have not been drinking and using for very long?

2. Why was it so important to change everything in my life?

Beauty Lost, Beauty Found

Jessica Overwise

First I have to say that there would be no glories at all to speak of, if I had not become sober. I was on my way to being incarcerated for the rest of my life or buried because of alcohol and drug abuse. This last August I celebrated 34 years of sobriety, thanks to a Higher Power and the unconditional love and fellowship I found through Alcoholics Anonymous.

I had been working as a casting director in the film and television industry. This position brought me into contact with hundreds of actors daily. At the end of a day of casting I would feel deep loneliness because I didn't feel connected to any of the human beings I had just interacted with. I drank to dull the pain of alienation. However, my world completely changed when I surrendered my drinking and using and chose life over death. My health improved dramatically, my ability to form relationships began to heal and grow. Today I have an extended family of literally hundreds of brothers and sisters; for an only child who grew up with two alcoholic parents, this is a miracle. There are so many glories to relate, but one of the most important to me has been the gift of being able to experience beauty again. It was something that had been burned out of my psyche from too much alcohol and drug use.

A chance meeting with an artist in New York City opened me up to a world I didn't even know I had lost.

Since I was a visitor in New York, Kevin suggested that I might be interested in seeing the exhibit of original sketches of Dutch artists, including Rembrandt, on display at the Pierpont Morgan Library. I had mentioned to him that I was never able to understand or appreciate paintings, even so, I was willing to visit the gallery. He instructed me to look at the sketch of an unknown Dutch artist and then look at a similar subject matter by Rembrandt, oxen over the bridge, that sort of thing. I did this several times and wondered what was so great about these drawings. Back and forth from the lesser artist and to Rembrandt's work. All of a sudden, something happened. I was able to comprehend the difference between the artists. Then I saw and experienced the genius that was and is Rembrandt's. It was an opening, a movement to another dimension filled with light. I was so touched that I quietly started to cry. The opening grew and I spent the rest of the day going to as many galleries and museums as possible, weeping almost aloud, while standing in front of Van Gough, Matisse, Renoir and many more masters of painting and art. I could see and feel the great works, as I had never been able to before. What a gift! I would never have been able to embrace this magnificent opportunity if I had not been clean and sober.

I live across the street from a national forest in the Pacific Palisades, California, where I take my daily hike. The other morning while walking and listening to my iPod, making sure I was exercising correctly, I was planning the day ahead, in other words, a very busy mind. Suddenly, out of the blue, a young fawn appeared in front of me. This had never happened before. The deer and I made fleeting but significant eye contact. My right hand flew to my heart and I held my breath at the sight of this wonderful creature. At first I thought he was moving slowly but it was the grace and elegance of his movement and the proud way he held his head and chest that caught my breath. A moment fixed in time. I whispered, "Oh my God! What beauty!" In an instant he disappeared, but I was brought into the present filled with awe.

Another gift I dearly treasure is being able to be quiet and meditate. My mind was so filled with negative thoughts and fears that I could not sit still with myself for any length of time. Today, I look forward to the times I can be alone to feel the presence of a deep and abiding faith that has grown slowly over the years in an inner sanctum I had no idea existed. This faith has led me to a freedom I had been searching for all my life. It brings with it the desire to forgive myself and everyone in my life for everything.

Another great gift, perhaps the greatest is that through sobriety I learned to love, others and myself. Today I am blessed with the most delightful intimate relationship I have ever known. I never thought in my life that I could ever form a healthy relationship with someone special. Indeed, without sobriety, that would have been impossible.

Sobriety has washed away the barriers between creativity and myself, between others and myself, and most importantly, between my creator and myself, which I choose to call God.

Today I am able to create my own art. My love for photography has enriched my life beyond measure. I now work as a professional photographer who photographs paintings, sculpture, and people.

The truth is that today I look upon life itself as a work of art and all of the beautiful people in my life as my family. I am grateful.

> "Beauty is truth. Truth beauty, that is all ye know
> on earth and all ye need to know."
> —*John Keats*

Biography

I started out in Stratford Ct. and New York City with a desire to be on the Broadway musical stage. I did perform in summer stock and on Broadway. However, my alcoholism showed up and I gave it all up to work behind the scenes. I moved to Los Angeles and became a casting director – helping many others achieve their dreams in film and television. After thirty years of casting, I started photographing and writing for the local papers. I have gratefully found an art that I seem to be good at and love. Along with the most wonderful friends and partner, this is my life today, thanks to sobriety.

Discussion/Reflection Questions

1. Are you willing to concede in your inner most self that you have a problem with alcohol and other drugs?

2. Are you willing to entertain the possibility that you have been out-of-control?

3. Are you willing to being open to a new you and a new way of living that is spiritually based?

Back Under the Sun

Alexander Popovich

If someone asks me what sobriety has given me, my answer would be simple and straight – **All** ! I am obliged to sobriety for changes in my life which I could not even dream about when I drank. Gradually, but surely, it gave me a new life, a family, the country where I reside, and a job. But the main change has been my new vision of life. To better understand what I am talking about, it is necessary to recollect who I was and what happened to me when I drank.

I come from a country that no longer exists anymore on the map of the world; I am from the USSR. I am sure that if, in June 1988, I had not come to a meeting of the first Alcoholics Anonymous group in the USSR (in Moscow, Russia) called "Moscow Beginners," I would not be alive now today. By the time I went to that first meeting, I had lost my family, changed places of work thirteen times in four years, and spent time in alcoholism treatments of Soviet "narcology," which then included taking medicines and injections, receiving deliberate verbal humiliation from staff, doing hard labor in prisons, working in a foundry, and helping with disposal of dead bodies from a psychiatric hospital where I was once placed. But the main thing I lost was myself.

I lost interest in everything, except for alcohol. I was a liar and dodger, constantly without money because I spent almost all of my salary for repayment of alcohol-related debts and spent the rest for new portions of alcohol. It is a shame to recall it, but at that time, I considered it a waste to spend money to buy myself new underwear because it cost as much as a bottle of wine. Obviously, the wine appeared to me much more important. I thought since nobody can see my underwear anyway, why spend money to buy any?

Alcohol gradually became the most important thing for me

and I submissively satisfied its whims. To me it was a shame to make eye contact with people because I did not know if I'd been drunk the previous day. I was literally pursued by small, but numerous trauma-bruises, the broken nose, burns, traces of scratches and grazes on the face.

But especially, I was ashamed of my shivering hands. I knew very well that only some dose of alcohol could help me, but I was afraid to drink during working hours because I was afraid of shameful dismissal. But one time, after a night of heavy drinking, close to noon the next day, the last grams of alcohol left my body, and not only did my hands shiver, but so did the rest of my body. A black chasm was opened before my eyes, and I felt that my heart had gotten off from its normal rhythm. I gave up all fears of shameful dismissal, left the building where I worked, and went to the nearest café where I could drink a shot of cognac or a glass of wine. While waiting in a small line, I decided it was too early for a shot of cognac, but a glass of dry grape wine would return me to life and help me survive till the end of work when I could really drink. When it was my turn, I greedily looked as the barmaid poured me this glass of wine and put it on a counter. I wished to take it, but I immediately understood that I couldn't do it because the shiver in my hand worsened as I was lifting my hand to the glass. I understood that I might simply spill all the wine, so I could not drink it. (Or, I could take a glass by two hands at home and pour wine in myself.) I whispered to the barmaid, "I shall return soon." I departed to a corner of the dining hall area. I was sweaty! I was shaky.

I humbly approached a single man who ate at a table and addressed him, "Excuse me, I beg you to help me! Do you see a glass of wine on the counter there? It is mine. I cannot take it as my hand strongly shivers. Could you bring it to me here where nobody can see me?" This man looked closely at me and unexpectedly asked, "Are you a right-handed person or a lefthander?" "I am a right-handed person," I answered, not understanding the significance of this question. "Then go and take it with your left hand." At first, it seemed that he scoffed at me. But he added: "Try it! If it doesn't work, I will bring that glass here as you ask."

I rose and slowly went to the counter. I saw only my glass. To drink this wine was the most important thing in the world for me at that moment. I cautiously stretched forward my left hand. It shivered, but only one-thousandth times as much as my right. The man was right! I took the glass with my left hand, brought it to my mouth and, knocking it against my teeth, swallowed its contents. My God, was I happy during that moment! I am alive! Moreover, it appears, I am not a terminal alcoholic. I just have to take glasses with alcohol by my left hand and all will be OK! In a week of my experiments with the left hand, it began to shiver even worse than the right one. I recollect this case and I can only imagine to what degree alcohol must have by then poisoned my brain. I had literally lost the ability to think normally and rationally.

Now I have been sober for many years. First of all, sobriety has probably given me Freedom: Freedom from alcohol and Freedom to be myself. It is not a shame to me anymore to make eye contact with people because now I remember what I did and promised yesterday, the day before yesterday, the weeks and months ago. I am not ashamed of my hands, which can do now the most precise work. Confidence and power have returned to me. Today I know what I want, and it not a shame for me to have those desires. I speak what I think, and I do what I speak. After divorce and separation from my first wife and son, and having passed my fortieth birthday continuing to drink, I believed that love of a woman and family happiness would never be granted to me. Fortunately, I was wrong, and my sobriety has rewarded me with this happiness. Never during my drinking times could I have dreamed that I would be included on a mission of sobriety across the USA in April of 1989. I could never have imagined that my two friends and I in recovery in Moscow, would be invited to the USA to share our experience, strength and hope with recovering alcoholics in the USA, and that we would learn from them a science of recovery.

The road of sobriety led me to my future wife, who has followed her own road of recovery. Sharron and I got acquainted in Los Angeles in April 1989; in August she arrived in Moscow, Soviet Union, for three weeks. At the end of this visit, I made a proposal and she accepted it. We became husband and wife on a snowy afternoon in Moscow in December of the same year. We certainly had some fears. How can we, people from two countries that were recently opponents in the Cold War, live in peace, love and contentment? But political disagreements of our leaders have been much less important than universal values on which we have based our sobriety: love, mutual respect, care and readiness to come unquestionably to each other's aid. Together Sharron and I look in the same direction, and have the same dreams and desires. We wish to stop killing ourselves with alcohol and to construct new, promising, mutual relations, based on sobriety, support, trust, and spirituality. We found each other. Our Higher Power worked, having helped us find each other on the opposite sides of the Earth. We have common interests, our desires about a sober and happy life coincide, and certainly we have loved each other every day. It was necessary to tell our parents and relatives in the USA and the USSR. They welcomed our union and have accepted us with open embraces. If God will permit, in the following year, Sharron and I will celebrate the 20th anniversary of our life together. Since 1990 we have resided in Los Angeles.

I have visited Moscow practically every year since then, where I meet with family and my sober friends. Sometimes passing by "my" old liquor stores in Moscow, I notice the same people are standing at them. It is "my best friends" then with whom I had drunk. Some of them are in the same place. Nothing has changed there, where the main value is alcohol. Only sometimes, one of them asks me: "Do you remember a certain person? He died two (three, five and so forth) months/years ago." I recollect this person, I wish the peace to his spirit and I recall how the sober life frightened me in those years. Somewhere subconsciously I felt, that all my interests, and all my life spun around a bottle. All in my life: friends and recreations, parties and sports events were associated for me with the use of alcohol. Sometimes wine, sometimes beer, and sometimes vodka. The bottle of alcohol I imagined as the main axis of my life, around which hopes of various areas of my life rotated. I was afraid that if this axis were removed, my life would lose its grounding and predictability. I recollect how comfortable I had felt then, together with these drunks who now seem to me unhealthy, flabby, and fat.

The understanding comes to me that then I simply was afraid of a sober life where it is necessary to be fair and to be responsible for my acts. I recollect, that in those days I practically never had money in my pocket. I almost immediately spent it for beer, vodka, wine, and sometimes various household, perfumery, or medical liquids which served as substitutes for alcohol because they cost much less than alcohol. Now it seems to me, that Higher Power deliberately destroyed all my money so that I could not buy a lot of alcohol that would poison me and accelerate the end of my life. In fact, the average life expectancy of a man in the USSR is only 58 years, because of alcohol and tobacco abuse. It became evident that the great majority of men did not live old enough to receive a pension. Now, when I am sober, I always have money in my pocket. At any moment I can buy as much alcohol as I want. But it is not necessary for me any more! Now I have other interests and desires. And probably Higher Power, seeing these changes, is not afraid anymore for my life and well-being, and allows money to be in my pocket. Now this money doesn't go to the destruction of my health and mind, but quite the opposite, to their restoration and maintenance.

I have visited the fitness club on a regular basis since 1993; I buy myself sportswear and socks, vitamins and sports food supplements, books and magazines for a healthy way of life. In 2006 I had triple-bypass surgery. Just after the operation I started to engage in fitness exercise with only one desire: to gradually develop my repaired heart to enjoy my sober life. Now I feel even better than before the operation, and with great desire I go to regular training to maintain my fitness. I like to be sober and healthy!

As I already mentioned earlier, my recovery became possible after my arrival to the Program of 12 Steps. The concept of the Higher Power or God as we understand Him, is one of the core components of this great Program. But I had lived more than 40 years of my life in the Soviet Union where I was very far from God. For me it was the greatest obstacle during recovery because I didn't understand God in any way, moreover, had been negatively adjusted to this word. I wasn't alone. My friends in the group, also grown on Soviet anti-religious propaganda, had the same feelings. Despite these difficulties, all of us were full of enthusiasm from our so long-expected sobriety and ready to work under that Program which gave real results. Our group "Moscow Beginners" then experienced a period of intensive growth. At almost each meeting two to four beginners came in, and the premises where we held our meetings became too small for our group. In the Soviet Union in those days, special permission to use other premises could be received only in a local state office. One day, at the end of 1988, I, as the secretary of our group, went to a meeting with a Soviet official to discuss obtaining a bigger place for our meetings. I tried to explain briefly to this official what A.A. is, and why we needed a larger place for our meetings. The authority figure listened to my information with obvious interest and goodwill and then said, "Well, what you do with alcoholics deserves encouragement and support. But understand me correctly, in order to give you new premises, we should know the principles and the purposes of your organization, and also a report of what you are going to do there. Can you provide such information?" I with pleasure put on his desk the text of 12 Steps that well explained our principles, purposes, and what we were going to do. The official slowly and attentively read the first step: "We have recognized, that alcohol has subordinated us to itself and that our lives became uncontrollable." His reaction was positive. The text of the second step puzzled him: "What is this force, mightier than your own, which can restore health?" He asked his question, but not listening to my explanations, had passed to Step 3: "We made a decision to turn our wills and our lives to God as we understood Him."

"What God is there? I see that you are just one more sect!" he exclaimed, "Please don't bother me anymore!" Our conversation was over. I was very much frustrated, but somewhere in my heart, I agreed with him. It seemed to me, that such a good business should not be connected with God. Later I described this talk with the authority figure to my friends in our group. The decision was born right there: We have to adapt the Program of 12 steps to our conditions, having thrown out God. Everybody agreed with this decision...except for one member of our group. He was an American who lived then in Moscow and helped in the creation of our first group of A.A. in the Soviet Union. This man passionately exclaimed, "You wish to throw out the main thing from the Program which is the principle of a Higher Power? Without it, the Program cannot exist!" He tried to convince us, "The 12-Step Program today works in more than 120 countries around the world and everywhere steps and traditions are the same! Even in South Africa where there is a clear split between black and white, at meetings of A.A. members sit together, and share their experience, strength and hope in spite of the color of their skin!" We tried to explain to our American friend, that Moscow is not South Africa, and we know our culture and the historical traditions better. We know what will work in the USSR. This hot discussion lasted more than an hour. In the end our American suddenly concluded, "Well, I shall agree with you, but only when instead of the phrase "God as we understood Him," you offer something of equivalent importance and relevancy for each citizen of the USSR that can correctly work in your culture." We were happy. "Certainly, we shall select such a concept easily," with readiness we answered. It seemed to all, that we could quickly and easily do that.

As soon as our American friend left the room, we began to offer the variants: "Mother," "The Native Motherland," "Nature," Someone even shyly offered, "Communist Party," but we all understood that all of these offers did not compare with words from the Program: "God as we understood Him." We discussed this until late at night, and then we agreed, that for a couple of days up to our following meeting, everyone would think about new variants from which we would select the best one. We departed to our homes.

I tried very hard to find a meaningful substitution, but found nothing suitable. For those days I came to understand that nothing can be stronger and more considerable than the concept "God as we understood Him." There was a weak hope, that someone from my friends would be more successful. When we met before the following meeting, nobody offered new variants that could be more significant, than that classic phrase. This was the end of our attempts to prove to ourselves and to others that the universal concept of Higher Power wouldn't work in the USSR. We silently admitted our defeat. This case had broken my aversion to God, and for the first time I had thought about other laws of life, than those I knew before. I have been well educated, and as an engineer-mechanic studied and used laws of a material/physical world in life and work: the law of Gravitation, the laws of Newton's mechanics, the law of conservation of energy, etc. without any doubts and did not demand explanations. Why couldn't I admit that there are also other laws of life?: The laws of kindness, human attitudes, gratitude, the importance of a positive outlook on life? I very much would like to leave forever the horrors of a drunk existence and to pass to another life that is full of harmonies, happiness, kindness and peace of mind.

I tried desperately to break through a wall to get to the next room, which seemed to be full of light and happiness. In my anguished efforts, suddenly someone spoke to me, "Why are you doing this useless work? Simply take one step to the side and enter there, through the open door. It is a much easier way to get what you want." And I took this step. And then I took another. I accepted the concept of a power greater than myself. New principles and ideas about life entered into my life. I began to try to leave my old understandings and to use my new ideas about life. Results encouraged me. It seemed, that someone much more wise and more strong than I began to direct my life. I have felt uncomfortable inside when I heard the word God, but the words Higher Power pleased me. I tried to apply humility, where I undertook struggle earlier, began to turn problems and fears over to my Higher Power, and learned how to live in the here and now. The understanding has come to me, that someone stronger and wiser conducts me in life. This Higher Power sees the entire picture of my life, and with tact and with love helps me to go on the foreordained way.

I recollect how hard I suffered when I divorced my first wife and our 12-year-old son. I then really believed that my life was finished and did not see any way out from that deadlock where alcohol led me. I was simply destroyed by our family separation. Only now I understand, that then it was necessary for me to pass through all of those challenges and leave them behind because ahead I had sobering up, new love, new family and relocation to the USA. Because of those challenges, when some years later in my new sober life Sharron appeared, I was ready (emotionally, spiritually and legally) to spend our lives together. Problems in life can be like pictures: If you come too close to a picture, then you will see only ridiculous and unclear botched work. Gradually, when you start to move back from a picture, ridiculous botched work will start to change and make sense. You can completely appreciate the beauty of the artist's creation only from an appropriate distance from the picture's surface. This is the same way I started to understand my problems and difficulties. All of them are rough strokes on a huge and fine picture of my wonderful life, which was mastered by the Creator. So I have come to humility and gratitude – two major qualities that have changed my life. Also I came to understanding, that I am not the God, and my opinion is only just one of many, instead of truth in the last instance. Sometimes it seems to me, that earlier I went to a blossoming field. The sun shone, birds sang, flowers around smelled sweet. But I did not see anything around and was concerned only by the momentary troubles. Suddenly, I fell in a deep, dark hole with musty water at the bottom of it. Only in this fetid pool did I suddenly understand how it was good above. I began to try violently to get out and move upward. I clung to wet clay ledges, strained with all my strength, trying to move ahead and upward to the desired purpose. But, one awkward movement and I again slid to the bottom. But, I persistently continued the attempts and eventually got out to the surface.

How happy I am to appear again under the tender sun, among the birds and colors. The picture around is the same, but I am another person now. I removed muddy glasses of indifference and negativism. Delight and pleasure of existence have flown over me. I am filled with huge gratitude literally for everything around: for these extraordinary bright colors and the blue sky, for wonderful melodies of birds that

I see. And I feel all this with each new beat of my heart. I have again returned to the world of happiness and pleasure, but appreciate all of this much more because I had dreamed a lot about it in that crude and dark hole. It seems to me now as if it is the maximum pleasure. Delight of life! I am blessed to return! All of this became possible only because I have ceased to poison my body and mind with alcohol. Sobriety is the key word to my pleasure in life!

Biography

Alex was born in Moscow, U.S.S.R. He earned his high-school diploma, completed military service, and got a MS (Mechanical Engineering); he worked 21 years as a technical designer in Moscow, U.S.S.R. He married and had a son. However, his drinking gradually started to cause problems with his career and family. Progressing alcoholism was destroying his life; Alex and his wife divorced after a 12-year marriage. His drinking forced him to change jobs every few months. He became a frequent patient at various alcoholism clinics in Moscow. Unfortunately, he did not have progress in recovery. In June 1988, quite by chance, he attended a meeting of the first A.A. group in the U.S.S.R.. Since then, his life has changed dramatically. He got sober, and about ten months later (April 1989), Alex was included in a small group of recovering Soviet alcoholics to visit the United States. During this trip, Alex met Sharron. They got married in Moscow in December 1989. Alex and Sharron have resided in Los Angeles since 1990. Alex completed college courses and has been a Certified California Addiction Treatment Counselor and Certified California Gambling Counselor. He works in two treatment centers in Los Angeles, California.

Discussion/Reflection Questions:

1. In the past, why was Alex afraid to have a sober life?

2. Why did Alex and his sober friends have difficulty accepting God in the 12-Step program?

3. How has Alex accepted the concept of Higher Power?

The Avenue of Miracles

Loretta Roth

To most of us the word 'miracle' seems to be a magical word. It anticipates good and affirms the presence of a spiritual power that can change something adverse to something healthy and rewarding. Growing up in an alcoholic home, I lived my life in constant fear, hoping for a miracle that would bring peace and happiness to our family. That miracle never came. As I grew older, I discovered that the path of our lives creates the avenue through which miracles can happen! We look for miracles and indeed, it is the looking, the very expecting, that opens our lives to them. Sobriety would become my "Avenue of Miracles".

I learned that in questioning or judging (as I was prone to do) people, places, things or situations, that I was questioning God's work. Everything is in God's time and when I find fault, I'm actually faulting God. This led me to experience one of many miracles:

I was on a plane coming back from Seattle, Washington after being at the International Convention of Alcoholics Anonymous. I noticed the man sitting across from me had long hair, a hat turned backwards, a coat that was apparently much too big for him as was his shirt. I decided right then that this certainly was not the type of person with whom I would want to strike up a conversation! I purposely avoided eye contact when I knew he was looking over at me, and then I remembered what the tenets of sobriety had taught me about judging. When he leaned forward a registration card from the convention slipped out of his breast pocket. When I looked over at him he smiled and I said, "You've been to the convention. Did you enjoy it?" He seemed to light up when he explained how he came to be there. It seems that some of the men in his Men's Group meeting got together and pooled their money to pay for his flight, his hotel and his registration. When I asked where he lived, he replied, looking down at the floor, that he was a homeless man, that one of the fellows had loaned him the coat he was wearing, another the shirt and yet another the hat. It was the first time he had ever been on an airplane or slept in a hotel. He was so very proud! We continued to share all the way back to the Ontario Airport. I offered to give him a ride to wherever he wanted to go but Willy said that the guys were picking him up. I saw his group as we disembarked, and felt joy and thanksgiving at having been able to share in this moment and experience the miracle because of my sobriety.

Sobriety and its teachers helped me to change my thinking and perceptions allowing the "Avenue of Miracles" to appear. I grew to know a God of my understanding that surrounds me with love, kindness and patience. I wanted to experience the miracles, the rich fruits of life, to stop hurting, to move into comfort, peace and confidence where the rough places are made smooth. I was able to do this by being *willing* to grow along spiritual lines, by staying close to my sponsors and their direction, by studying the Twelve Steps and working with others, and by believing that everything is possible through my Higher Power. The miracles just keep happening.

One of the most precious miracles was that of my father making his commitment to quit drinking when he was eighty years old. He loved to come to my home for a visit and while he was with me I offered to take him to a meeting; it was to be the first of many meetings. My home group was loving and kind to dad. They welcomed him with open arms inviting him to come back. My father was a proud Irishman who loved his whiskey, laughter and jokes. His favorite joke was about Pat and Mike and goes a little like this: Pat says to Mike, "I'll be going to meet me maker soon Mike and I'd like to ask a favor of ya. After they be putting me in the ground, would you be going out and buy a bottle of the finest Irish whiskey and pour it over me grave?" "Sure" says Mike, and

I'll be doing that for ya, but would you mind if I strain it through me kidneys first?" God kept dad with us for another two years before taking him home. After his funeral we had a beautiful reception, but I missed my brother and I couldn't find him anywhere. Finally he walked through the door and I asked him where he'd been. He said he had gone out and bought the finest bottle of Irish whiskey money could buy and went to the cemetery, poured it over dad's grave and said "Here is the finest bottle of Irish whiskey money could buy dad, but we don't find it necessary to strain it through our kidneys any longer." What a blessing, that could never have happened but for the miracle of sobriety!

One of my finest miracles happened when God placed an angel, Faith Strong, into my life. She asked me to join a group in taking the message of recovery and sobriety to the Soviet Union through an organization called Creating a Sober World, which she created for this purpose. How beautiful the people of Russia and the Ukraine are – so many touched my heart! They wanted health and happiness for their children just like we do. Touched by their stories, I thought whether you are surrounded by the lace curtains of America or the iron curtains of the Soviet Union, the devastation that alcohol does to our lives and the lives of those we love is the same. We took that message over for the first time in April 1986 with government approval and many others and I have returned a number of times to continue carrying that message. In 2007 I was privileged to return to Moscow to represent Faith Strong, who was unable to make the long journey, to celebrate the 20th year of Alcoholics Anonymous in Russia. My heart overflowed with joy and thankfulness as I walked into their convention arena and saw over 3000 Russians, old and young, celebrating their lives in sobriety.

Maybe sobriety doesn't make the world go round, but for this alcoholic, it is what makes the ride on the "Avenue of Miracles" worthwhile!

I've recently gone through a divorce that didn't have to be filled with anger and resentment because of what I have learned in sobriety. Instead I was able to walk through a painful experience with dignity and grace.

Each day is a fresh opportunity to love myself and others a bit more and to judge myself and others a bit less. On a daily basis I know that each time I can do something unselfish, that is spiritual, and when I make amends to those I have offended or harmed, that is spiritual. When I can remember to speak of the good in another person or reach out to give someone a helping hand, that is spiritual. When I see the beauty of nature or listen to inspiring music, that too is spiritual. In the simplest of things, God allows spirituality to be discovered and performed. I would not have the spiritual life I have today without having traveled the path of addiction to sobriety.

As I continue to grow in sobriety, so too continues my "Avenue of Miracles."

Biography

Loretta Roth was born and raised in California and has lived in many parts of the United States.

She received her certification as an alcohol and chemical dependency counselor from the University of California at Irvine.

Her love of life and of people have taken her to many parts of the United States, Canada and Europe.

Loretta has been blessed with twenty-six years of continuous sobriety. Sobriety date: February 5th, (best 5th I ever had) 1982.

Discussion/Reflection Questions

1. What "miracles" are you looking for?

2. How might sobriety change the way you perceive yourself?

3. How could sobriety change the way you view others?

My Expanding Consciousness

Larry Shrimp

There is a dear person that I am so very blessed to have encountered. She has accomplished much in her lifetime, but, it is more than her many accomplishments that draw me to her. It is the way Spirit shines through her to me. You can imagine how I felt when this wonderful lady asked me to write a chapter for this book. I felt honored and amazed. I never considered myself a writer nor did I believe I had much to say. I had shared my life at meetings, but writing or public speaking were not in my past list of accomplishments.

I, however, was so excited about this invitation that I felt compelled to tell many other people. I rode this horse called excitement for quite a while and then it was time to produce: Time to collect my thoughts. Time to start writing. I thought about the task. Why was my life so full of happiness and free of the bondage of liquid spirits for so many years?

In order to get focused, I asked a group of newly recovering alcoholics and drug addicts living at my sober-living homes to anonymously submit questions for a person with ten years of sobriety. I was astounded at the quality and depth of the questions. They are listed below in their entirety:

> How do you keep being sober exciting?
>
> They say willingness is the key to begin sobriety. Was this true for you?
>
> What do you struggle with today that you also struggled with in the beginning?
>
> How important is being of service to your sobriety?
>
> What role does sponsorship play in long-term recovery?

What is meant by spiritual awakening?

What do you do when you are bored?

What tempts you most to use again?

What is the key to long-term sobriety?

Do you still have cravings and urges?

Do you consider yourself recovered or in recovery?

What is the number one thing that helped to keep you sober for ten years?

What was the last straw?

Did you know that you didn't have one more in you?

These questions got me started; they made me think about my life. I believe that in the following most of these questions are addressed.

My 84 year old mother lives just next door. A few weeks ago, in my usual jovial manner, I asked her how she was enjoying the beautiful day. She said she was having the worst day of her life. Wow! Over 80 years on this planet and she was having the worst day of her life. I said I was sorry to hear this and moved on to my next adventure that day. This has left an indelible spot on my mind. This could have been me and for a while it was my way of looking at the world. Being raised by my parents, I could and did absorb many of their values and ideals.

At another time, a few years ago, my father, my mother, and her brother and I were having lunch together and the conversation led to their father. Her brother had made some lighthearted comment about their dad. My mother snapped at him saying, "So you think that so and so was funny." I then learned that their father was an abusive alcoholic and that my mother for all these years was still carrying the hurt she felt as a child and the hate she thought he deserved. She had never forgiven him or herself for those childhood experiences.

In the third and last story about my parents, I wasn't even present. My daughter, who since she was a young student has known that her dad is gay, was talking with my mom and dad and mentioned something about how badly gay people were treated in some situations. My mom informed my daughter that she felt that those people ought to be treated like everyone else.

Fear, mistrust, bigotry, hate and general disdain for life on this planet can be harbored. My low self-esteem developed from life with my parents. They were more than displeased that I was one of those gay people and one of those alcoholic people. We don't even need to mention that I was divorced, against organized religion, living with another man, not a millionaire and not even an elected official.

I, like others, had to go a long way to dispel the awful way I thought about myself and become someone that I could love.

The middle years of my life were spent somewhat productively. I owned and operated an electrical contracting business for 35 years and just 15 years into that business I started a small manufacturing business making beautiful landscape lighting fixtures. I bought a house, nice car and many toys. I married and we had a daughter together and then divorced. I did all this while actively drinking and can't remember feeling joy during these years.

Just over ten years ago several things happened in close proximity: my daughter expressed how much she cared for me, a drunk driving arrest left me with debts, a suspended license, drunk driving school and an AA court card. Life just didn't seem worth living and the spiral down pointed to the bottom. I could see where I was going and it wasn't good.

I made a decision to change my life and embraced AA with all the gusto and enthusiasm of a man clinging to a rope that was preventing him from entering the pits of hell. I have never regretted this decision to change my life. Every minute, every day, every week and every year that passes allows more joy and happiness to enter my life. Through working the steps of AA, I found I could enjoy life without the aid of liquid spirits. I reconnected with the God that I had previously denied existence. I enjoyed the presence of another person in my life, my AA sponsor. It was not always easy working with my sponsor. We met every week for six months and diligently read and discussed each of the AA steps – as well as checking in on how my life, AA meetings, work, family, etc. were developing. We continue to support each other and ten years later we sort of sponsor each other. We have much common ground to stand on as we are both alcoholics.

Attending AA meetings and functions, as well as having a sponsor was such a treat in my life. For the first time I was able to communicate with others in a totally honest manner. I didn't need to lie or put on airs. There were times when I was scared, specifically when it was time to share. After all I was raised to believe I was not good enough and up until this time had no other input to change my mind. With each meeting attended my anxiety decreased and this fearful little guy became less afraid.

Through these AA years, I was able to build a new philosophy of life for myself and it was all about the above and especially those famous 12 steps. In the beginning I had to read and understand the steps. Some call it working the steps. Then, after understanding the steps, I needed to practice the steps and with practice I found that they worked. They always work.

Finally and to this day, those steps have become a way of living. I have the AA philosophy of life. I have recovered. No, this doesn't mean I can drink like a gentleman again. I'm not cured. That ship has sailed; it will never sail again. What it does mean is that I no longer think about having a drink every minute, hour, day or week. I no longer romance the feeling one associates with a drink and the cravings have disappeared.

Continuing with my AA experience, I have been blessed with the sponsorship of three wonderful men. They have taught me so much in life. The first taught me about the importance of sober living and its relationship to lasting recovery. The second demonstrated how we should never stop giving back and helping new people find recovery. He still works in the recovery industry. The third, a talented artist who had covered his talent and productivity with a veil of substance abuse, is now again a wonderful productive artist. He has shown and sold his work from the Festival of Arts in Laguna to other galleries around the country.

For the first seven years of AA I was amazed and satisfied with the spirituality I found in the program. When I entered the program I was a professed atheist. Within only a few weeks and because I was willing to have a different life, the door opened and I found the God of my understanding. At first, I didn't love God. I was still afraid of God. As the years passed, I grew to love myself and God at the same time. The spiritual hole that I was insanely trying to fill with liquid spirits was filled with Spirit and Truth.

Around year seven I felt the desire to broaden my view of spirituality and I started looking outside of AA for more spiritual adventures. After visiting several places of worship, I found a place that felt like I had come home. The teachings of this organization meshed well with all I learned in AA and my inner feelings of how a life full of joy and happiness should be.

Sobriety first and then my world started to expand and it has never stopped expanding. First I'm on a spiritual path that is unending. The more I read, study and learn about my life as a spiritual being, the more there is to know, experience and love. I have taken every class available and embraced the teachings of this spiritual center as I embraced AA. I recently became an intern practitioner and will be entering ministerial classes soon.

I found a way to be of service and express my unique talents in this organization. I was given the opportunity to become the manager of the little bookstore at the center. Happily I chose to say yes. I have been trusted to do my own thing and its been a rewarding experience. I first tore out walls, opening up the store so merchandise could be easily viewed and accessed. I expanded the selection of books and gifts. The greatest joy, however, was making use of the blank empty painted walls to display art. Yes we now have an art gallery. It is a great area for attendees to show their art as well as local artists from the community. This enhances the overall beauty of the spiritual center and the center benefits from the sale of art.

Having made a recovery from my addiction, I have been able to support other alcoholics and drug addicts that have chosen a life free from their unwanted attachments. I expanded my home to allow sober-living space for five recovering men. I purchased another home a block away and turned it into another sober-living environment for eight recovering men and recently leased a third home for an additional eight. I keep close to the recovering community through this adventure.

Sobriety has allowed me to experience life to its fullest and my spiritual connection has allowed me to be a human being not just a human doing. I do, however, enjoy doing.

Sailing is a love and in my first year of sobriety, with all the money I was saving from not using, I bought a small sailboat and named it Serenity. It has a home in Dana Point Harbor.

I love to do new things, have new experiences and push my life to its limits. I recently crewed on my sponsor's sailboat, his first competitive race. I knew I would be in for a lot of excitement and probably get yelled at for not making his boat go faster. I wasn't disappointed. I was yelled at but I was only doing the best I could and no one was yelling at me in anger, just exuberance.

I took piano lessons when I was in my pre-teens. I never became a concert pianist and I don't even attempt the classics anymore. However, I still love to play the piano and recently, I am playing with more expression and feeling than ever. I'm still involved with the landscape lighting company that I recently sold. I assist with design and sales. I get to do what I love without the obligation of doing the work. I just bought a new bicycle, and really love the bike trail from downtown to the beach. The parks along the way are great places to rest and meditate.

Everyday, when I wake up I enjoy contemplating what I will experience that day. There is more and more and more because I am open to new experience in my life.

The story of my glories of sobriety would not be complete without mentioning two of the most wonderful parts of my life. First, my life partner Chris. We have stood by each other over the last 15 years of our lives. When we met we were both practicing alcoholics and the first few years were full of drama, broken dishes, broken dreams and broken hearts. When I got sober the arguments ended. It's so hard to fight when one sees the futility in war. Just four years ago real magic happened. Chris decided he was through with drugs and alcohol too. What a joy it is to have the clouds, formed from the vapors of alcohol, lifted, and to see the truth in each of our lives. We try to make all decisions that directly affect us both, together. It might take some extra time and effort and a lot of discussion but when we make decisions together we end up with truly beautiful results.

As mentioned earlier, I have the most beautiful family and it resulted from my meeting a wonderful woman. Due to my sexual orientation, the marriage was brief. However, we have been friends from our first meeting to the present time and have enjoyed loving and mutually supporting each other and our daughter on all of our lives' journeys. She was the first person to whom I made amends at the beginning of my sobriety. I will always be grateful to her for presenting us with the beautiful child we call our daughter. I am happy to be gay but to be gay and father a child is truly magic.

My daughter married the most loving, caring and outstanding man. My ex-wife and I dearly love him. Our daughter has given birth to a most wonderful child, our granddaughter, Zoë. Her second child is due to begin her human experience very soon.

The joys of my sobriety are more than I could ever have dreamed. There has been a great shift from darkness to blessings too numerous to count.

I would like to close with the words of my daughter as they were written on my last father's day card:

> "Happy Father's Day Dad. We all love you so much
> and truly appreciate the person that you have
> become. You've turned out to be the best father I
> could have ever asked for. I hope it's a great day
> and that we have a hundred more of them.
> Love, Denise."

Biography

Born June 8, 1941

Lives with partner Chris in San Juan Capistrano

Sobriety date July 17th, 1998

Electrical contractor retired

Loves people and animals and life

Loves sobriety

Discussion/Reflection Questions

1. How important is change in your life?

2. Do you feel stuck?

3. What would you change to have more fun in you life?

The Gifts of Sobriety

Ruth Stafford

It's been a good weekend and the end of another beautiful
August day. I watched my grandchildren play at the beach
while my daughters beat me at Scrabble under the beach
umbrella. I am filled with gratitude for sobriety as I reflect
on my day that included breakfast with friends, lots of laugh-
er with the grandchildren, and planning the week ahead.
My weekly calendar is filled with useful interesting work and
play. Before sobriety, a perfect Sunday like this was impossible. If Sunday started out well, which meant that the hangover was under control, it inevitably ended badly. How great
it is to wake up on Sunday morning without feeling as
though I had a bad case of the flu!

Sobriety, the freedom from alcohol and drugs, has opened
me to the wonders of the world and the knowledge of my
inner self. When I shut off feelings that I didn't want, such
as fear, anger, guilt, and shame, by drinking or taking drugs, I
also shut off joy, aliveness, excitement, love and caring. Life
today is Technicolor rather than the black-and-white repeti-
tious bad movie my life had become. Often, I am propelled
into the Present. So much of my life before sobriety had been
spent in the past with regrets, or fantasizing a grandiose
future that could never have been realized when I was drinking. One of the benefits of sobriety is the freeing up of time
and energy that were spent drinking and recovering from
drinking. There are so many interesting places and people to
know, useful activities, and fascinating experiences. I want to
live life in its fullest with gratitude and appreciation. I do
most of the time.

Sober life is a fascinating path that is not always easy. I
walked through the deaths of my parents and best friend.
Sobriety allowed me to deliver the eulogy and to mourn
appropriately for those loved ones. Walking through a bout

with serious breast cancer last year resulted in many gifts that I was able to receive because of being sober. The support of many friends, some who walked through breast cancer themselves, was invaluable. Knowing that breast cancer, like alcoholism, can be arrested gave me hope and reassurance. Just as living sober has been cause for examination of my life, so has this recent brush with cancer. I have become less busy and find more time for family and friends, and for being of service to others. I am more thoughtful in considering the best use of my time and energy. Many opportunities for growth present themselves every day.

After a failed alcoholic marriage and several sober single years, twenty-four years ago I was blessed to meet and marry a wonderful man. We have never seen each other drink. He has a great sense of humor. We laugh a lot. In our senior years both of us continue to grow in understanding and love; we share our sobriety. Our home has held many fun parties. We enjoy opera, classical music, theatre, movies and travel. In sobriety, we have traveled the world. When we travel sometimes things go wrong and nerves get frayed. One of us will then decide that we need to have a meeting. We center ourselves with the twelve-step format, even if it's only the two of us in a hotel room in a remote area. We have done this in cruise ship rooms, in a mountain cabin in the Andes of Venezuela, on dive boats in the South China Sea, and in a hotel room in Bangkok. The two of us even had a topless meeting in a very hot hotel room in the jungle of Ecuador. It works every time in our letting go of the annoyances that sometimes go with travel plans.

We started scuba diving together before we were married and have been all over the world diving in the Caribbean, Egypt, Southeast Asia, Mexico, Canada, and the Pacific Islands. The high that I get from diving is far better than any feeling that I had drinking. Breathing slowly, being close to weightless, and surrounded with incredible beauty is thrilling. At the same time it is a focused meditation. One of our best trips was a scuba trip with nine other sober divers to Cozamel. We wrote ahead to charter a small boat to take us out every day, calling ourselves the Sober Divers. Arriving there we discovered that the owner of the scuba shop was also sober as well as a dive master. So she took us out where we had fellowship, fun, and diving. Before jumping in, we all held hands and said the Serenity Prayer.

I have a close loving relationship with my two daughters, a relationship that was very difficult through their teenage years. They were following their genetic heritage of alcohol and drug abuse. My greatest joys occurred when each daughter surrendered to recovery. They have been clean and sober now for many years. They say that my example of recovery eased the breakdown of their denial and inspired their desire for a sober life. We have traveled together to Italy and Mexico sharing laughter, food, and the sights of Venice, Florence, Oaxaca, and the Yucatan. My younger daughter, who lives on the East Coast, and I have great times in New York City going to the theatre, sightseeing and shopping. I am very aware that these kinds of fun experiences are possible only because of our sobriety. One daughter's husband, whom she met in recovery, and my other daughter's boy friend have also been sober for a number of years. Family gatherings are loving and fun filled.

When I started recovery, I was treading water in a Ph.D. program that I couldn't finish. Sober, I was able to write my dissertation and finish my Ph.D. in psychology. After teaching at the University for several years, I passed my exams for a clinical psychologist license. This allowed me to work in the field of chemical dependency treatment and recovery. I love this work. When an alcoholic, a drug addict, or a person addicted to prescription drugs becomes and stays clean and sober, the change that occurs is miraculous. No other type of patient the mental health professional treats results in the miraculous change in a life that sobriety brings. It is very rewarding to witness and be part of that change. Although I see hope and a good life return to many of my addicted patients, I have also had to grieve many who were not able or willing to make that change. It always feels as though they have refused a wonderful opportunity for a bountiful life.

The greatest gift of sobriety is finding and growing a spiritual relationship with a Higher Power that I call God. It was practically impossible for me to let go of control of persons and things that are uncontrollable before sobriety. I don't know why because I wasn't any good at it. Without a consciousness of a Higher Power, it felt to me as though people and situations I deeply cared about would fall into an endless abyss if I let go of control. With faith that there is a greater plan that is unknown to me, I am able to give up playing God myself. I often am faced with the fact that life is what happens when I'm making other plans. And it often is better than I could have imagined.

Today I am comfortable being me most of the time. I have come to accept myself as an imperfect human being who can regard mistakes and character defects as a challenge to grow and behave in ways that are consonant with my core values of love and service. It is good to be free much of the time from the fear and anxiety that I had consistently when I was drinking. Today I have choices as to how to live life. When I was drinking, my life seemed to unwind like a bad movie that was happening to me. I felt helpless which I handled by blaming others for my predicament while, at the same time, beating myself up for it. Today I recognize that my life is my responsibility and that there is no solution to a problem if I do not recognize my part in it. One of the great benefits of sobriety is that rather than playing roles and changing behavior and attitudes to fit in with the persons and situations in which I find myself, I am myself in most all situations. It takes so much less energy to be consistent and true to who I am rather than attempting to hide my self-hatred and please others. I feel that I am much more the person that God intended me to be and for that I am eternally grateful.

I have recounted only some of the blessings of sobriety. There are so many more. I surrendered to the search for sobriety and recovery after a terrifying incident. One Friday evening after an afternoon of martinis, I saw a vision of myself in the mirror of the ladies room. I saw an old lady with deeply etched lines in her face – lines of pain and dissipation. I believe that I saw a vision of where my life was headed: getting old beaten up by life and chemical dependency. Today I am 72 years old, healthy, happy, and useful. If I hadn't embraced the opportunity of sobriety 36 years ago when I saw so clearly where I was headed, I would have missed out on the only good years of my life.

Biography

I live and have a clinical psychology practice in Laguna Beach, California. My professional career as well as my personal life has been focused on understanding and treating chemical dependency. This has included research, writing, teaching, lecturing, treating and twelve-step work, all of which have contributed to my continuing growth. My greatest blessing has been the sobriety of my two daughters.

Discussion/Reflection Questions

1. What would you like your life to be in five years with regard to family, work, intimate relationships, service, spirituality, health, etc.?

2. What pleasurable and fun activities do you want to pursue in sobriety?

Stay for Another Miracle

Susie Stern

"Don't leave before the miracle happens." These are the words that I kept hearing in the rooms of AA, and these simple words are what kept me coming back for more. It showed me just a sliver of light, a sliver of hope that helped me to believe that just maybe, just maybe there was a miracle out there waiting for me.

I came to AA when I was fifty years old and had been divorced for twenty years. I divorced when my two boys were one and three years old, and I had to go to work full time to raise them. I would like to say that I was a good mother every night when I came home from work. I want to think that I put my boys on my knee and read sweet stories, or that I asked them about their day. I want to think I was their calm voice of reason, and that I could tell them that everything was going to be all right. But instead, I came home from work tired and angry, shouted orders, and put them to bed early.

I also would like to think I was a popular girl and had many dates and love affairs. The reality was that I had hardly had one decent date in all those 20 years. The one big romance I did have was when I was 50 years old. It was my last chance at love. I had believed that he was the one. He came to me complete with parent approval, and I knew we would be married happily ever after.

I was wrong. The relationship ended abruptly and I ran for cover. This man's rejection of me was like a death sentence. It was a crushing blow to all of my dreams, and I gave up on love and happily ever after. I came running to AA, took my seat, and surrendered completely.

I felt like a wounded animal and came to AA for a miracle. Everything I had tried to do to live right had led me to the same lonely place. My disease was my loneliness and the feeling that I was worthless and unlovable. I had spent twenty years moving from apartment to apartment and job to job chasing miracles and thinking I could find the perfect husband and the perfect job on my own. I didn't think I needed anyone to tell me what to do or where to go. I was in charge.

But I was wrong. I needed help. I needed to change my thinking and my behavior. I needed teachers and people to guide me and support me. I needed something in my life to help me calm down and to help me feel safe and loved. My instincts told me that for all of this to come to be, I would need a lot of miracles.

My first miracle was getting a sponsor. She called me "Hon" or "Honey" and made me feel loved. She became my calm voice of reason and told me every day that everything was going to be all right. She told me to memorize the Third Step Prayer and to say it every night until I went to sleep.

I had been having a hard time getting a good night's sleep. I had given up drinking and smoking, and had begun eating a whole can of roast beef hash fried in butter just to relax and get to sleep each night. Of course, this didn't help, so I memorized the Third Step Prayer instead. Each night when I went to bed, I lay in the dark and said this prayer over and over a million times over until I went to sleep. Every time I came to the part that said, "Relieve me of the bondage of self", I would relax a little more and get a good night's sleep. I would feel better each day and knew I had experienced a miracle and the beginning of a new healing.

The Third Step Prayer helped me to know God and to surrender my will to God's will. God became my constant companion and my wise counsel. I trusted God and went to Him with all my questions and problems, and I never stopped thanking Him for my new start on life.

Even though I was getting a good night's sleep, my anxiety

and anger and fear were still alive and well inside of me. They worked me over on a daily basis, and I ended up in a deep depression. I could hardly get up out of bed. I slept and ate and walked and slept some more. I began to have a dream, and this dream kept coming back to me over and over again. The dream was a painting of Santa Barbara. I had raised my boys in Santa Barbara, and now my boys were grown and gone. The dream brought back fond memories of raising my boys. The dream became bigger than the depression, and finally I got up and went to the art store. I brought home some art supplies and created my first painting and surprised myself. The painting was of the Santa Barbara Mission, the Courthouse, sailboats in the sea, beach umbrellas on the sand, and a million little white houses with red tile roofs held together by thousands of palm trees. It was colorful, and happy and naïve. I didn't know I had "colorful, happy, and naïve" in me, but the proof was in the painting. I hung that painting in my apartment and painted some more.

The painting helped to connect me to life. I started to feel loved and was learning how to love back. I loved everyone's stories. I admired the courage it took for AA people to get up in front of a group and tell the truth about how hard life had been for them and how they had been graced by God's love. I learned to laugh and to cry and how to love and appreciate everyone in AA.

I learned to have compassion for everyone, especially for my ex-husband. I learned how much I had hurt his heart when I just blithely took his children away. I learned how I had hurt my children's hearts and my own heart when I divorced and, in turn, kicked out our family's very foundation for feeling loved and safe. I had single handedly broken our family apart, and I didn't know how to put it back together again.

I apologized to my ex-husband, and he let me know he was fine and had a good life and that he thought I had been a good mother to his boys. The boys also thanked me for being a good mother and said they would always love me. I didn't feel like I deserved all of this goodness and love, but it made me feel better.

My next amends were to myself. I had left my marriage without giving my ex-husband a chance. I had been self-will run riot and didn't think it through. I had left on the coattails of another man thinking he would be a good husband. He was not a good husband, and I spent the next 20 years looking for my safe place and someone to love.

My first attempt at amends to myself was to find a husband. I went to an old friend, who I hadn't seen much in 25 years. I had always loved and admired her, and she had been married for over forty years. She knew what a good man and a good marriage were all about. The two of us had lunch, and I asked her if she knew a good man for me.

She did, and I began to date Fred. He was easy to date, because we simply went out to dinner once a week and were always back by 8:00. When he asked me to go away for a weekend, I stopped in my tracks. I didn't want romance with Fred. I wanted to go out to dinner once a week with Fred and get back by 8:00. So I said I would have to think about it.

I was still raw and unsure of my instincts. They had never led me to love and security in the past, so why should I trust them now? I went to my sponsor and to AA sisters for wise counsel. Then I went directly to God. I asked God about Fred: "Why am I dating him and should I stay or should I leave?"

God said that I had never been treated this well by any man in my entire life and that I needed to appreciate that. He said, "Fred is very nice and that I wasn't so nice. God told me to be nice. Treat him well and see what happens."

I was nice to Fred that very day, and that very day I fell madly deeply in love with Fred. This was my miracle. I began walking on air and life became easy. I had never known a love like this. Fred made me feel safe and loved. He took me places I've never been, and he was kind to my boys. He respected me for my recovery from alcoholism and loved all of my AA friends. He introduced me to his Jewish culture and I found how similar it was to my Presbyterian background, and how similar it was to AA. We would go to the High Holidays and then to the Presbyterian church and sing God's praises. Then I would take Fred to an open AA meeting, and he would be touched.

We built a dream house made of wood and glass that looks out onto a sage covered mountain. This is the mountain that I look to every morning to give my thanks. It is where I have my finest talks with God and with my parents, who had passed away right before my biggest miracle happened.

My parents never knew Fred. They only knew me as a divorced woman in the world feeling lost at sea and alone. They knew me as a drinker and a smoker and angry and rebellious, and they worried about me until the day they died.

I believe that today the spirits of my parents are alive and well on the mountain, and that they see how happy I have become. They see what a nice man I have married and how well my children are doing. The mountain is where I go each day to find my serenity and love and where I go to thank God for all the miracles in my life.

Now that God has made all my dreams come true, and I have experienced such life altering miracles, it's time for me to grow up and live life well. I'm learning to talk more slowly and softly. Instead of that old angry reactive voice that I thought would get me through life, my voice is softening, and I am becoming a calm voice of reason. This is having a good effect on my relationship with my husband, my children, my sponsor, my sponsees, my ex-husband and his wife, all my friends and family, and especially on me. I am no longer that lonely woman lost at sea.

Today I have a great big family that does many things together. We sing and dance. We go to the beach and have family vacations together. We meet for Passover and Thanksgiving and Christmas, and I've learned to cook a good meal. After I broke our family apart so many years ago, and after we all ran so far away from each other for so many years, we have all found our way back home. We all have a family of our own. We all live in the same town, and we all share a family kind of love.

Everyone in the family has at least one painting of mine on the walls of their home. This is my redemption. This is what helps me to know that I have been forgiven, and that I can love without bounds. I can love without conditions, and I can be loved back.

I have learned that AA is a wonderful way to live, and as long as I live right, the miracles never stop. Whenever I think that I might be cured and can drink like a normal person, I say to myself, "No! You're not normal. You're an alcoholic. Don't drink. Live well, and stay for another miracle."

Biography

I was born in 1940 and was raised in San Marino, California. I joined AA when I was 50 years old and got an education in life. I learned that I was an artist and surprised myself. I learned to appreciate everything creative and artistic, and now I paint almost every day. My art connects me to life and enables me to share my joy with other artists, friends and family.

Today I am 68 years old, and every day I am grateful for my husband, two sons and their wives, three stepchildren and five grandchildren. I have been married for ten years to the man of my dreams and am living happily ever after.

Discussion/Reflection Questions

1. What is it in life that would make you feel safe?

2. What is it in life that would make you feel loved?

3. What do you need to change in yourself in order for you to begin to live life well?

Alive, Awake, and Free

Faith Strong

Comparing being sober with not being sober is like comparing night and day, dead and alive, insanity and sanity, war and peace. The non-addict cannot possibly understand what it's like for a recovered addict to live with sobriety. It's a huge thing for us, where as it's as natural as breathing to a non-addict. And even though I've had many years of sobriety it's a challenge to write about it.

When I thought about describing my sobriety, three words jumped out at me: alive, awake, and free. That's the way I see myself today.

Being alive at the age of eighty-six is a blessed gift. It never entered my mind that I would live this long. And without sobriety I would certainly not be writing this nor would I have envisioned this book. I am so grateful to be alive! When I think of all I would have missed over the years – for example, being there for my children. I remember when I first thought of creating a yearly family reunion. There had been much separation, many negative judgments and misunderstandings, because of the divorces and alcoholism in our family. I wanted my family to heal as I was healing – to heal just by being together: playing, sleeping, sharing, laughing and crying. It was a labor of love finding a house big enough to accommodate us: six adult children, their spouses and children. Someone, I can't remember who, found one in a local desert community. We were uncomfortable and awkward with one another at first but by the end of the weekend love was all that was there. Every year we had a reunion at different locations, always concluding the weekend with a sharing circle (including the very young grandchildren). I recall that one reunion was held in Washington State close to Whitman College where my youngest, Deborah, was graduating. We all danced at her graduation party. What fun we had!

These reunions continued for many years. Today they keep in touch with one another, know each other, and even with their differences respect and love one another. Without sobriety none of this would have happened!

As for my grandchildren, oh what a tragedy if I had missed seeing them grow up. They have turned out so exceptionally well: healthy, talented, smart, beautiful human beings. All seven of them! How I adore each and every one and glory of glories they communicate their love for me. Could sobriety have brought me any better treasure than this? I have one great grandchild, still a toddler and another on the way – I've been with Taj (he lives on Maui) and look forward to meeting his sister.

But the very best benefit from sobriety is being here and being alive to support, and express my deep gratitude, appreciation and love to them and for them.

Being alive gives me everything. The opportunity to learn, to grow (yes, especially when you are eighty-six!), create. Very often when I am in the shower I belt out an old song, "I love life, and I love to live!" Of course, I have the usual aches, pains, and worries that come with aging but when I contemplate the alternative there is no contest.

Being awake – oh yes! I love waking up each morning – no matter what! This is my pot of gold at the end of the rainbow. (I do hope that my "after life" has something comparable.) Waking up every day without guilt, without shame, without wondering what I did or didn't do the night before, with an anticipation of the waking hours ahead; waking up to doing a lot or to doing nothing – each being equal in importance. Being capable of "smelling the daisies," enjoying my breakfast, and just being content and at peace with myself and others.

This was a long time coming. I was so painfully shy, self-involved, and unhappy most of the time that being comfortable with others or myself was out of the question. At any event, gathering or meeting I would always arrive late and leave early or preferably not go at all. As for "smelling the daisies" I didn't even see the daisies much less smell any! And breakfast was unfamiliar, sleeping through it being the better choice.

Today it's just the opposite. In sobriety I've had lots and lots of requests to speak in front of large audiences and to small groups. One big one comes to mind. I was being honored by the Hunger Project in New York at their important Africa Prize event – a formal dinner of two thousand people. They came from many countries and included Presidents, Ambassadors, leaders, journalists and celebrities. I was instructed to keep my acceptance speech to ten minutes, to write it down and have it approved by the Hunger Projects' Director. What an order for a recovering addict! Some of my family were present and lots of friends but also lots of strangers and this was not an A.A. meeting. I prepared my little talk (I kept thinking that it was after all just a little talk). I dressed from head to toe in black (for protection). They had me scheduled between the entrée and dessert. I was terrified! The Dias was elegant with seated U.N. dignitaries, celebrities and leaders of the Hunger Project. Joan Holmes, President, was the first to introduce me (after I had been assisted to the steps of the stage). Then, Valerie Harper, the actress, introduced me and helped me to the stage. I was being honored for my long time commitment and contribution. I stepped up to the podium, after receiving a gorgeous crystal sculpture, and began with "My name is Faith Strong and I am a recovered addict of 33 years. My drug of choice was alcohol," totally forgetting my written speech. I then shared my love of the Hunger Project and what it meant to make a commitment and to make contributions. I was really surprised at the lengthy applause. I was awake and able to do this without a drink or a pill.

Freedom! What a powerful and gorgeous word. And today miracle of miracles, I have it! Without sobriety I was in shackles and chains, unable to think, unable to feel, unable to move. With sobriety I am free to think, to choose, to create, to feel all of the emotions, to express them and be free of fearing criticism. Today, with glorious sobriety I am free to be comfortable with myself, anywhere and with any one – I enjoy my own company. I am free to imagine, to see a need and be able to contribute to it. Without sobriety I was unconscious that there was a need. My children suffered the most from this maternal negligence. I was there physically but my mind was "out to lunch." My heart was with them but not my listening. I did a lot of pretending by cooking, giving gifts, making promises and apologies. But I was too self-involved to hear, to see, to feel their needs – their real needs! Today I can intuit a need and certainly am capable of responding to one when they request it. As I became healthier and healthier I began seeing my neighbors' and the worlds' needs. And not always, but often I try to respond.

With sobriety I am free to follow instructions: Like those of my doctors or my family; like reading maps (forget folding the darn things) and even the instructions "To Open" on a box or package. I was too impatient, too ego-centered. A.A. calls it "self-will run riot." This willingness to follow instructions has come with having the patience and teachability that I never had.

I guess the two accomplishments (outside of relationships with others and myself) that are the most dramatic examples of my sobriety are founding A.A. in Russia and publishing three books. Having a vision in 1982 to create A.A. in the Soviet Union, making a commitment to have it manifested and then creating the first open government approved A.A. meeting in the Soviet Union in 1986, was one of the biggest thrills in my sober life.

This story is too long to tell it here but I can truthfully say that Russian A.A.'s seeing me as their founder is really hard to accept and believe. They had their 20th year celebration of Russian A.A.'s existence in Moscow in August, 2007. Three thousand Russian A.A.'s attended!

My other big accomplishment has been writing. Everyone can write, has a story to tell. You just have to believe it. And you have to be clean and sober. I am more alive, awake and free when I am creating. The hardest thing about it is to begin. Writing is fun, painting is fun, cooking is fun. Inspirational words like these supported me: "There is only one you and if you don't express your idea, your imagination, your talent, it will be lost to humanity forever."

I am also free to have fun! I don't need or want a pill or a drink to have fun at a party, a wedding, a dance, a celebration. But best of all, I am free to be me – to enjoy my own company because today, it's good company most of the time. I am free to keep my word and to be able to count on me.

Last but not least, none of the miracles of sobriety would have been born without the support and principles of A.A., my family and friends, transformational seminars and spiritual leaders. Recovery gave me the courage to go through the healing process of breast cancer, and the courage to accept that I'm nearing the end of my life. Thanks be to God I'll be clean and sober.

Biography

I was born in Kansas City, Missouri on July 21, 1922. I am a recovered addict of 44 years. I celebrate my sobriety every day with my six children, 7 grandchildren, 2 great grandchildren, friends and neighbors.

I was born again the day I got sober: September 16, 1964.

With sobriety I re-discovered my creativity – expressed through painting, writing and visioning. Publishing three books and bringing A.A. to the Soviet Union in 1986 brought me great joy and fulfillment as did manifesting my vision for this book. What is next for me is honoring a request from my kids to create a CD singing the songs that I have composed.

With sobriety, even at 86, it just gets better.

Discussion/Reflection Questions

1. Am I willing to make being sober the #1 priority in my life?

2. How do I support my commitment to sobriety?

3. Do I know that I am capable of creating a clean and sober life?

Getting Out of Yourself

Tom Whelan

In the last month of 1965 I was desperate for a good night's sleep. One would think, consuming over two quarts of vodka and/or scotch, several Librium throughout the day along with some Secondal, it would be easy to sleep all night. I would wake up in a couple of hours, pace the floor, drink more, take more pills, pass out again for a few more hours: I had lost my wife of twelve years and lost private meetings with my two little boys, ages ten and eleven. Somehow the judge involved, didn't approve of my taking my two boys to Sunday Brunch at my favorite bar, The Cork and Fork. I had recently been discharged from a mental institution where I was put for taking a hundred Secondal sleeping pills followed by a considerable amount of scotch. I was about to be charged with passing bad checks at The Cork and Fork and the neighborhood liquor store. I knew that I could not stop drinking, nor did I want to. I knew though, that I could not go on living the way I had been for the last few years.

At Mass, at St. Paul the Apostle Catholic Church, on Christmas Day, I knelt at the rear of the church and begged God to "Grant me some peace." Two days later, I believe He heard my prayer. After my morning drinks, I noticed a quart bottle of Scotch, which I had purchased just the night before, was almost empty. I remember remarking to myself that it was a lot of scotch to be consumed in less than twelve hours. That night I wound up at an Alcoholics Anonymous meeting at a hall on Ohio Street in West Los Angeles.

I attended meetings there for about ten days. I still didn't believe I could really live without drinking, but I went to the meetings anyway, fortified with enough booze to avoid shaking, wanting to appear relaxed, so I would fit into the crowd and not be obvious to anyone. One Tuesday night in the first week of 1966, I was seated at the meeting. When they asked for "newcomers" I didn't move. A stranger sitting next to me raised my hand. For some unknown reason I allowed him to do that. When the meeting was over, I got up enough nerve to talk to one of the people who seemed to be in charge, the secretary of the meeting. I asked for his help. I asked him how it was possible to stop drinking and stop taking drugs. He stopped what he was doing, took me aside. He gave me some actions to take to not drink the following day. I suppose I was so desperate that I listened to his suggestions. He told me to simply get up in the morning, get out of the apartment and drive to the Santa Monica beach to spend the day walking, drinking Karo syrup, eating Hershey bars, walking up and down the shore. I didn't drink that morning. I made it through the afternoon and went to my first meeting sober and drug free.

I was shaking and sweating all the time. No one seemed to notice. Everyone was most kind to me and they invited me to join them at a coffee shop after the meeting. I did that after most of the meetings and repeated this almost every night for about two years. During this time my wife and I got back together again. It was great being home with the family after almost a year. My wife was none too happy with my being gone every night at meetings. But, for the first time in about fifteen years, I was sober. The adjustment was difficult for both of us. She neglected to attend Alanon meetings. She was seeing a psychologist at the time and didn't feel it was necessary to attend meetings. She did come to some A.A. meetings.

I suppose it was about eight or nine months later. We had not been getting along. I remember leaving a Friday night meeting absolutely crazy. When I was in my car I noticed I was crying, then laughing, then both at the same time. I went for a long drive and ended up at the beach. I couldn't really put my finger on what had me so upset. I drove by my sponsor's house. I woke him up and he invited me in. After we talked awhile, he suggested that it was time to do an inventory – a fourth step. Since I had spent a number of years with a psychiatrist, I really didn't see the point of hashing all this out again, especially writing it out. Being a Catholic and spending time in the confessional, I felt I had done enough soul searching. I believed that I had spent much too much time delving into my mind and my past. My sponsor saw it differently.

I proceeded to write my inventory. I was as honest and forthcoming as possible. When it was completed, I met with my sponsor and did a fifth step. Even though I was concerned that he would think badly of me, I put my feelings aside and read the whole thing to him. He listened and didn't seem bothered by any of it. As it turns out, he had heard the same stuff from many other people over the years. Now that I have been sober a long while and have sponsored dozens of men over the years, I can see how boring most of our stories can be. None of it is very earth shaking.

At my sponsor's direction, I found a quiet and private place to get down on my knees and take a sixth step following by reciting the seventh step prayer. I have incorporated that into my set of prayers that I say often every day.

For my eighth step I had to list my many creditors, which added up to over $ 30,000.00. In the sixties that amount was insurmountable, so much so that I consulted a bankruptcy attorney. He sent me the forms to fill out and file. Though at first hard to understand, long-term members of Alcoholics Anonymous suggested, that if I indeed owed the money, I simply owed the money and that I would have to pay it back, no matter how difficult or how long it would take. It took me over eleven and a half years to settle these accounts.

I felt, to stay sober I had to clean up my life and that meant paying back all the people I owed. I had to become responsible in all my dealings.

Basically, I amended my life so that I maintained a clear conscience so I would never have to put any sort of poison, like alcohol or drugs, in my body again.

For the next seven years, I remained sober. I worked hard in my electrical contractor business. My father died in early 1970. Since we worked together and had a wonderful relationship, I was really lost when he died. As insecure as I was, running a business totally on my own, I simply used the A.A. program taking everything a day at a time, one job at a time, one customer at a time. I did the best electrical job possible for each client and I was moderately successful until the early seventies when a recession hit and work was very slow. Our marriage, never really good, was suffering. I discovered that my two sons, about seventeen and eighteen, were addicted to alcohol and all sorts of drugs. My wife and I argued over this and other issues. We agreed to separate and she filed for divorce. I moved my business and my life to South Orange County and built a moderately good business.

I was not aware that my wife was manic depressive or bipolar. About two years after the divorce, she managed to buy a .38 caliber pistol and shot herself. After an operation and a stay in a mental institution, she had been all right for the last few years. In light of this, I felt guilty for what had happened to her. Yes, I had made amends to her years ago, but still I wondered if I had not been alcoholic, maybe things would have been better for us. Now that so many years have passed, I have learned to forgive myself and get on with my life.

I married again in March of 1979. My second wife was also a member of Alcoholics Anonymous. I was thirteen and she was nine years on the program. We had a good marriage although it only lasted until Christmas of 1985. Our entire time together was spent dealing with her breast cancer: seven operations, chemotherapy and radiation treatments. Not only were my two sons dealing with their alcoholism and addictions, but also my new wife had three daughters and a son with the same problems. Trying to keep a business going, dealing with all the family problems, supporting my wife with her serious health conditions, our life was far from dull. I am certain that our heavy involvement in Alcoholics Anonymous carried us through. We were invited to speak at A.A. conferences all over the country and locally. When death took her in December of 1985, I ended up in a depression that lasted almost a year. I was now twenty years sober and really couldn't enjoy my life.

On looking back, I had lots to be grateful for. Both my sons had found A.A. and both loved the program. Along the way there were difficulties: one was diagnosed with HIV and slipped back into addiction for a while. The other went through a divorce. For my part, watching my two sons struggle with their problems, I was grateful I had the A.A. philosophy well ensconced inside of me.

I married again a couple of years after my second wife died. We have been together for over twenty years. She also is in the A.A. program. We enjoy a comfortable life together.

Over these last 42 years, I have experienced many situations that would have beaten most men. With the aid of A.A. and my involvement with over two dozen men I actively sponsor, my life is good. Last year I had a four-way bypass. The help was enormous from the people in A.A. I have learned to keep active mentally, physically and especially spiritually. I plan to keep working in my business for some time. I workout in the gym five days a week and walk three miles on the beach on the weekends. My life is beyond full, thanks to what I have learned in A.A.

I would say that Alcoholics Anonymous has taught me to live in the now. My nature is to live in "the wreckage of my future." Staying in the present is the key. I also have learned to accept life as it comes. Life is really ups and downs – in any area. Accepting whatever comes gives me the serenity I have most of the time.

When asked what has kept me sober all these years, not only sober, but mostly comfortable and having a personal inner serenity, I have to believe it is my attempt to get out of myself. I have to face the fact that I am really mostly concerned with myself: my family, my business, my health, my finances. Really, left to my own devices, I am consumed with myself.

In Alcoholics Anonymous, I have been taught to get out of myself; make calls to people to see how they are, whether I care or not. Ask the guys how they are. What can I do to help them get through what they have to get through? In my electrical contracting business, naturally I am concerned in getting paid as much as I can, but instead, I adopt the attitude of giving each customer the best job I can and helping them solve their problems by installing or repairing whatever is needed.

At home, I do my best to see what I can do to make home life better for my wife. It seems when I think less about what I want, our relationship is at its best. My wife recently lost her mother. I supported her in her loss and all she was involved with: the arrangements with the funeral, the sale of the house and dealing with the family. Naturally, I was concerned with my needs, but I concentrated on her needs and did whatever I could to make it easier on her.

Maybe all this makes me sound like a phony. So be it. I really don't think it matters. I believe I have very little control of my thoughts or my feelings. I do, though, have complete control over how I behave – how I act. Strange as it must seem, when I act well, I feel well. When I feel well and good about my actions, the chances of my going back to those horrible days, before I found this new way of life, are slim.

So, I suppose, I will continue on this path. When my mind tells me differently, I will continue to tell it, "Thank you for sharing, but shut up!" and continue to keep laughing and seeing what I can do to help others.

Biography

Tom Whelan is frequently asked to speak at A.A. meetings and conferences – four to six times per month in his local area as well as nationally. He has been in the electrical contracting business since 1956. And, he has been sober for 42 years, beginning on January 6, 1966.

Discussion/Reflection Questions

1. What should you do when you have a craving?

2. How does living in the present moment help you live one day at a time?

3. How does serving others impact your ability to stay clean and sober?

The Wilder family wishes to Dedicate
this chapter to our Mom and Friend,
Pamela Floyd Wilder

Sobriety Runs in the Family

J.L. Wilder and Lyn Wilder

When I was born in Laguna Beach in 1973, I was the second child of two alcoholic parents. And for my sister and me, that was a wonderful thing. My parents had met and married in sobriety. They lived in the spiritual principals of a 12 step recovery program, and learned to walk through life together...sober. For my sister and me, we literally owe our lives – and the wonderful upbringing we had – to sobriety.

Growing up in a sober home meant that we had no experience with the alcohol-induced chaos, violence or drama that is common in alcoholic homes. Our parents were never drunk or hung over. There were no blackouts, no drunk driving episodes, no late night calls from police stations or hospitals. Our parents were active and loving participants in our lives. They coached our sports teams, were active in our schools, and showed up for the important moments in our lives...sober.

Our parents learned in sobriety that Love and Service are the basics to life, and they tried to live according to these principals. Mom was active in helping women in recovery. In 1977, at a time when there was a significant stigma attached to alcoholism – and particularly alcoholics who happened to be women – Mom stood up in a Jr. League of Orange County meeting and identified herself as a recovering alcoholic. As the room of women listened in stunned silence (not many women were willing to publicly admit alcoholism in 1977), Mom explained the critical shortage of rehabilitation treatment services for women suffering from alcoholism. She asked for the Jr. League's help and support in establishing a recovery program that would provide a safe place for women struggling with alcoholism to begin their recovery in dignity and grace. She got the support of the Jr. League, which allowed for the creation of a women's rehabilitation center in Orange County that has changed thousands of lives since 1977.

Dad also led an active sober life. Alcoholism brought him from a good family and loving upbringing in Kentucky to being homeless on the streets of Los Angeles. But he was able to get sober and put his life back together. In sobriety he was able to develop a relationship with a daughter whom he did not see for 9 years as a result of his active alcoholism. He met Mom through sobriety and started our family. And the two of them developed a deep and loving bond that enabled them to face life's challenges sober. Like Mom, Dad also devoted his life to serving others and lived an active life of sobriety. He was an active circuit speaker and spent many of his weekends away from home as he carried the message of hope and recovery to groups all over the country.

Of course, growing up in a sober home doesn't mean life will be perfect or that there will be no challenges. We had our fair share of difficulties, as all families do. The most significant of these challenges was when Mom was diagnosed with cancer in 1984. We've all heard it said that when things are tough you find out who your true friends are. What we discovered was that we had more true friends than we ever imagined possible. The close bonds that my parents had developed with a fellowship of recovering alcoholics became clear in our time of need.

That fellowship surrounded and embraced us with love and support. When Mom was in the hospital, they were at her bedside and in the waiting room. When my parents couldn't be at a big event for my sister or me, the fellowship was there for us. When Dad needed strength in the face of losing his soul mate of 19 years, they supported him. And when Mom passed away, they stepped in to comfort us and to lend us their strength.

While the benefits of growing up in a sober home were great, I was determined not to be an alcoholic. My parents were careful in how they handled the topic with my sister and me. They knew something we did not, that alcoholism runs in families. But they never told us not to drink. What they did say was: "Both your parents are alcoholics. This greatly increases the odds that you also will be alcoholic. We're not going to tell you how to live your life, but we think it's important you understand the risks."

But I didn't understand the risks. My response was something to the tune of: "Thanks, Mom and Dad. I'm a strong kid, I've got rock solid will power, and I have no intention of being an alcoholic."

Years later it became clear to me that I had not defeated the gene pool. Drinking increasingly became a problem and was having a negative impact on my life. The more I fought it, the worse life got. So I fought harder. I could conquer this just like I'd conquered everything in life. I'm a strong man. There may be alcoholism in the genes, but I grew up in a sober, loving and supportive household.

That stable home opened great opportunities for me, and I made the most of it. I worked hard in school and athletics as a kid which opened the door to an Ivy League college, which opened the door to Wall Street, which opened the door to an Ivy League MBA, which opened the door to a career in finance.

Then, one day, the doors all shut. I was a full-blown alcoholic, completely alone in my disease, and in desperate need of help.

As helpless and hopeless as I felt at that low moment, I remembered my parents and the sober fellowship that they were very much a part of. I knew that what was ailing me was alcoholism, and just as importantly, I knew that recovery was possible. I knew that there was no shame in alcoholism. It is not a moral question or an issue of restraint. It's not my fault, nor is it the fault of anyone else. I had an illness that I could not cure on my own. I needed help.

While I did fight it for quite some time (Who wants to be an alcoholic? Who wants to admit defeat?), it wasn't until I let go of the fight – and surrendered myself entirely to the notion that I had an illness that I could not conquer alone – that the process of recovery began.

My Dad and I recently spent a week on Cape Cod together, and we reflected on the gifts that sobriety has given us. There is no doubt that both of us have the disease of alcoholism. But more importantly, both of us lead active and healthy lives in recovery: In 2008, Dad celebrated 43 years of sobriety and I celebrated 5 years. Both of us have been fortunate in that we have turned our lives around after near fatal struggles with our disease. We have returned to healthy spiritual, physical, mental and emotional condition.

Our relationship has changed in sobriety. I no longer have to worry about hiding my drinking. I talk to him about my problems today, rather than pretending I have no problems. I don't lie to him and his phone doesn't ring late at night when I'm in trouble. I talk to him about the challenges I go through in life, and we are open with one another about the joys and sorrows, fears and emotions we each face. Our relationship has deepened, and a trusting and loving bond has developed that could not exist if either of us were actively drinking.

There is a serenity in both our lives that never existed before. The chaos and drama, the dishonesty and arrogance, the fear of impending doom that were so much a part of our lives are no longer with us today. I used to sleep until noon on

Saturday and Sunday, usually with a hangover and some combination of anxiety, shame and guilt. Today weekend mornings are my favorite time of each week. Dad used to drink every day, to the point where he couldn't function in life without alcohol. Today, it is a great feeling to wake up feeling refreshed, without the heavy burden of active alcoholism, and to be thankful and excited for the day ahead. That is a gift of sobriety.

Sobriety has given us the ability to live freely in the moment. While previously we lived our days focused on whom or what had wronged us in the past or what terrible event was waiting around the bend, today we are able to keep it in the day. We thank God each day for our sobriety and treat it as a gift. We believe that our primary purpose in life is to stay sober and to help others. There is a simplicity in that purpose, and as a result life is much simpler. When things get chaotic or challenges come our way – as they often do in life – we remind ourselves that our primary purpose is to stay sober and help others. That simplicity makes all else more manageable.

The greatest gift that we have both been given is a relationship with a loving God who runs the show. When I first got sober, there was no God or any form of spirituality in my life. Booze was my higher power. It was where I turned when times were tough or times were good. It's where I turned if I felt bad, if I felt I had been wronged, or if I felt the need to escape. Alcohol was my offensive and defensive weapon.

Dad's sponsor was a man from Laguna Beach named Chuck C. He used to talk about the ego of the alcoholic. He defined ego as "a feeling of conscious separation from". The ego was a wall we built, supported by alcohol, that separated and "protected" us from the outside world (God and our fellows) and our innermost selves. At the peak of my illness, alcohol had created a wall between me and the rest of the world. And now that alcohol was gone, the wall was beginning to crumble. As that wall came down, I felt exposed and filled with fear. How can I live without alcohol? What do I do with all these emotions and feelings and fears?

And that was where the "god thing" first played a role in my life. I was certainly no Bible thumper, and I was fairly skeptical if there was a God at all. But I remembered that spirituality was very much a part of the lives of my parents' sobriety as I was growing up. So I became willing to give it a try. Besides, I was desperate. So I started praying: every morning, every day, every night. The result of all this praying was that spirituality began to take on a meaningful role in my life. I have found that as the alcoholic wall of ego came down (as we believe it must for any enduring sobriety), spirituality has taken its place. Spirituality has become the answer to life's challenges.

Today, Dad and I try to lead a spiritual life. We try to do the right thing. When we pray, we don't ask God for a laundry list of things that will improve our status or our bank account. We ask for willingness and acceptance. We ask for humility. We ask for God to help us have a positive impact on those we come into contact with each day and not a negative impact. We ask for the strength to walk through what comes our way each day. We ask that God's will, not ours, be done. We ask for the strength to help others, and that we remember daily that our primary purpose is to stay sober and help others. We ask God to help us remember to keep it in the moment. To this day, the greatest gift we've received in sobriety is a new perception of a higher power in our lives.

Spirituality has become the guiding force in each of our lives. We believe everything in life is tied to the daily maintenance of our spiritual condition. One thing we have both learned is that while sobriety has improved our lives tremendously, it does not mean that life's problems completely go away. We still make mistakes. We have faced great challenges, separately and as a family. There have been financial struggles, relationship issues, conflict, the passing of loved ones. We have learned great life lessons in sobriety. We have made bad choices. But we have also learned how to walk through life's challenges sober.

Today we understand the importance of prayer and meditation and helping others. We have learned to watch out for resentment. We start by trying not to blame others but looking directly at our role in each situation. Prior to getting sober, we always seemed to be the victims. Others had always wronged us. Life wasn't fair. Today, we have learned to look at our part in every situation rather than focus on what others had done to wrong us. We have learned the importance of honesty, both with ourselves and with others. We understand the importance of being able to forgive others just as we have learned to forgive ourselves. It's not always easy. And we fail more than we'd like to. But we have learned to have a deep and enduring faith that no matter what happens, we can walk through it. We have developed the slow understanding of having faith in the process and then learning to turn that faith to trust. We trust that we will be OK. As long as we continue to do the footwork, to take the action needed to improve ourselves, we trust that things will work out exactly as they are meant to.

For Dad, family has been a great joy and gift of sobriety. Dad glows when he talks about his oldest daughter, who after finishing college and law school has been an attorney for over 20 years. She continues to be active in her professional life and maintains positions on several charity boards. Dad beams about his middle daughter, who having finished college has been a school teacher and mother to two beautiful sons. And he glows over his youngest too, and is proud to have watched me face this disease and turn my life around.

After losing his soul mate of 19 years, he has been able to pick up the pieces and continue on with life. Sober. He met another wonderful woman 12 years ago. They are now married and living a blessed life. She has two sons, one of whom is married and recently gave them a beautiful grand-daughter. Both sons are active in running the family business and very much a part of their lives today. He feels blessed to watch and to participate in the lives of all of his adult children. As he said during our week on Cape Cod together, "the greatest and most significant years of my life have been the past forty three years I've been sober. I thank God every day for my sobriety and treat it as a gift."

And I would agree with Dad on that one. The past five years that I've been sober have been the best time of my life. I have grown comfortable in myself. I have gained a willing-ness and an acceptance in life that gives me an inner peace that I never had before. I have learned to walk through life situations sober, often for the first time. I have renewed damaged relationships with family, friends, and coworkers. I understand today that there is no shame in having the disease of alcoholism; the shame is in not doing anything about it. And so I work hard to stay in fit spiritual condition so that I can stay sober and be helpful to others. I have learned to focus on the positive rather than dwell on the negative and to trust that everything in life is exactly the way it's meant to be.

A few years into sobriety I met and ultimately fell deeply in love with an incredible young lady. She naturally developed a peace and a serenity that I have to work hard to attain in sobriety. She brings a balance and a joy to my life that no one ever has before. She is the type of woman that I always dreamed I would fall in love with one day, but never thought would really happen. She is also the type of woman who never would have put up with my shenanigans back in my drinking days. But we have grown together these past few years and were married last year. She is a joy in my life, only made possible because of the sober lifestyle I choose to lead on a daily basis. Life is good. Sober.

Biographies

The Wilders: Both father and son contributed to this chapter. Lyn Wilder lives in Laguna Beach, California with his wife, Daneen. Between them, they have 5 children and 3 grandchildren. Lyn's son, J.L. Wilder, is recently married and is an executive at an investment management firm.

Discussion/Reflection Questions

1. How does alcoholism impact family relationships?

2. What do you think the authors mean to "live freely in the moment"?

3. What do you have to overcome to forgive others and to forgive yourself?

Gratitude and Grace

Loriann Witte

How do I feel about myself today after 21 years in recovery? I can sleep. I go to sleep at night, right out, without taking anything. Before getting clean, I would lay awake and suffer, thinking of my many insurmountable problems. My mind played movies every night in living color. I'd relive embarrassment and shame from the now showing selection of my mental movie collection. In the early months of recovery, sleep did not come easily. I was told I wouldn't die from losing sleep. Thank God I hung in there and stayed clean waiting to see that staying sober would change my life for the better. We have to give staying clean time, time to change us.

In active addiction my life led me. I just watched as things happened to me. All thinking was centered in the getting and using and finding ways and means to get more. The disease of addiction talked to me all of the time. "OK Loriann, you just stay high," while we go to divorce court. "You drive better drunk," so now we are going to jail.

Going to meetings and working a program has taught me so many useful skills. Some of what I hear shared in meetings teaches me what to do and some of it teaches me what not to do. It's all good.

If you are wondering what going to all of these meetings can possibly do for you, know that all of us had this same question. It's a new way of spending our time with people. It is healthy to be around other people who are in the process of making a difference in their own lives and the lives of others. The people in the meetings are talking about what they are doing to cope. As alcoholics and addicts we know plenty about the problems of life. We know all about what we do not want. Solution is the message of the program. Meetings are a life style. I go most every day because that is what I believe will keep me clean and sane.

Taking step 1 of the 12 steps made me realize I was powerless over drugs and my life had become unmanageable. Working the steps and going to meetings quieted down the voice of my dis-ease. I am now free to choose how I act and even how I think. I'm learning to put a positive spin on most everything. I feel so much better because of positive thinking. I declare myself as happy, joyous, and free.

For me, I feel that I have found my life's meaning. I roll through my life suiting up and showing up. I do my part as a human being. From the time I wake up in the morning, any time symptoms of the dis-ease start to come on me, I keep reminding myself to think, how I can be of service. The Big Book of AA says some symptoms of the disease of addiction are 'becoming bored, restless, and dis-content.' I know I have to watch out for these feelings.

Living ones life trying to make others happy is often a characteristic of the addictive life. While recovery is about being of service, and learning how to give, it is also about taking care of oneself so we have something to give. We must always replenish the well. We can't give away something we haven't got. There are paradoxes in the program. Stretching beyond our comfort zone is how we grow. We must be willing to be a little uncomfortable and try new things, but then find a way to be comfortable in this new action. We can be of service without trying to be who other people want us to be. We must find a way to be kind to others *and* ourselves.

Most of my life I was shy. More than shy I was afraid of people. I could only communicate by being rough and tough, or a desperate victim. In recovery I have been taught that my shyness was a kind of self-centered fear. My life was controlled at one time by the fear of what people would think of me. As I listened in meetings I came to understand that everyone spends most of their energy thinking about themselves and not so much about me. Raising my hand and sharing in meetings taught me that I do have something to say. The people in the meetings started responding to me differently when I was able to share new solutions. I was learning.

I'm not afraid anymore. My feelings of anger and rejection were based in fear. I got to take a look at these old feelings and events with a sober head. While writing my steps I came to know a lot of the unrest I went through was fear. Some of the 12 step writing led me like a road map. Writing the steps established a state of grace in my thinking. I went back over things and started to see that everybody does the best they can think to do in each moment, just as I have. What happens does not have to be judged as good or bad. Observing the passage of time and events without judgment is a gift of serenity. It is important to be slow to anger and quick to forgive. I began to forgive others; I have since then forgiven myself. I feel safe and sure. I love myself. I passionately enjoy being alive.

I have learned how to love myself so much, that I can love you and carry the message of hope in recovery. I've come a long way, baby. I don't know why I had to walk the crooked path. The why of the past isn't as important to me, as it once was. What I know is true is that my way has been made clear before me. The crooked path has been made straight.

As I write this story I have been married for 28 years. My husband and I have come a long way in learning how to be loving partners in peaceful co-existence. Through much trial and error we have come to know how to support each other's individual life experience without one life defining the other. I walk beside my husband giving as much love and respect as I can muster. When his walk is not a part of my highest good it gives me another opportunity to individuate and have personal strength within my self. In the course of a long term marriage (or even a new relationship) people don't always live up to who they want to be. My husband is my dear friend as often as I let him be and as often as he is able to be. I appreciate the times of love and support we have been able to share with each other over the years.

I married my drug connection whom I met in a bar at 6:00 A.M. We were married 6 years before recovery. Even after we got clean we were not always sober together. That's the way it is and this reality has to be acceptable to me if I am to know peace. All in all my marriage is the best part of my life.

In my years as a member of the recovery community I have seen many people come and go. It appears to be much easier to get clean than it is to stay clean. Only the diligent make it for any period of time. Meeting makers make it. An absolute joy is the miracles that have unfolded before my eyes. I know the ones who have come and stayed in the program. We share our lives together. By sitting in meetings with these people we do the "wed and the dead" together. It is said NA means Never Alone.

I have seen everything that could possibly happen to the parents and the children of recovery. Some couples stayed together, some did not. In my 21 years of recovery I have seen life find a way; the next generation is there, ready or not, life goes on. I know program kids who are so healthy they shine brightly. I know program kids who have died already. I believe the kids of those who stayed clean are innately better off than the kids of those who have continued in the struggle.

This is the life that I choose to live: I go to work; I go to meetings; I go to my church. I am not floating around the edges of the safety and happiness zones.

Relationships are my favorite thing. When I go to church, I make sure people know I am there. When I go to meetings, I most often speak up and share; I thank the speaker, and stay after the meeting to talk to people. At home, I talk on the phone to people who are not using and who want to help me in my recovery.

A large portion of my spare time is spent maintaining my spiritual condition; I listen to peaceful music so I can have some meditation. Good food, decorations in my clean house, walks with my dog –this kind of stuff keeps me together. My wellbeing is of top priority. Doing what is important to me in a way that I can feel good about myself makes it possible for me to stay clean and to serve others. Recovery has taught me that a gentle flow with life is what I desire; it is most reasonable to treat myself and others genteelly. We reap as we sow.

I went from a broken lost soul to a woman of power. What a transformative journey. Maybe your addiction story is similar or very different than mine. Getting clean and sober is possible for all of us. Getting clean and sober opens the door to changing our thinking. What I think about myself and how I think about others has truly changed. I have learned how to live walking the path of serenity and good will. For this I am grateful.

Biography

Loriann Witte is married to Pat. She and Pat used together and got clean together. They both work in treatment. At the time of this writing, they have been married for 28 years and are best friends.

Loriann has a house in San Juan Capistrano, California, where she enjoys walking her dogs, and sleeping with the kitties. She is active in the 12-Step community and loves her Church of Religious Science and Agape friends.

Discussion/Reflection Questions

1. "I am not my story." "I had to release my addiction to story." What do these phrases mean?

2. How important is it to ask for help – to keep asking for help – then to make the very best use of the help you receive?

3. What does it mean to "walk the path of serenity and good will?"

Twelve Steps to Freedom

Rita McCabe (formerly Wyatt)

As I began to think about writing this story my mind became flooded with memories and events that I had over the past thirty-one years, and last week, for the first time in many years I had a drinking dream. That dream took me straight back to all the feelings I had before I received the gift of sobriety on the 18th of April, 1977.

I had feelings of humiliation, guilt, shame, anxiety, anger, fear, etc. etc. The only relief was to drown them with alcohol. At that time, that was my only solution. Today my life is so different that it is difficult to recognize the 1977 me.

Sobriety began with the acceptance and awareness of my alcoholism, not an easy step by any means. It took a great deal of courage to raise my hand that first time and many times after, to say the words, "I am an alcoholic." At the same time, and for the first time I could remember, I was being validated and supported by strangers, and they appeared to be genuine. I had a very hard time with the "God thing;" I had grown up with a punishing and angry God. No matter, I was accepted by the group and it was suggested to me that I could use anything that had more power than me. For the first year I chose the group that I called my home group. Gradually, and using the wisdom of the group, I eventually found a very loving and forgiving God of my understanding. I learned the difference between "religion" and "spirituality." This was a crucial step for me.

I began to take direction, attend meetings, read the literature, be of service, and lo and behold I began to feel better. I was invited to sober social events and the belief I had of never having fun again began to disappear. I have had more fun in the sobriety years than I ever could have imagined. I have friends today that I got sober with. Some of my good friends

153

threw a 30th Anniversary party for me, and 150 people showed up for that event and completely overwhelmed me. In 1977 I spent most of my time feeling alone and lonely, passing out on the couch, with the help of alcohol almost every night, in front of my three teenagers who did not know what to do with me. Today, when I have a problem, I can pick up the phone day or night and call any number of people, talk about the problem and get into the solution. I rarely feel lonely.

I was 43 years old when I got sober; I had started drinking at the age of 14. I also left school at that age and did not have a high school degree. For many years in sobriety I blamed that on my father and the way I grew up in an alcoholic family, which gave me the opportunity to play the victim role. I was ashamed of the fact that I had so little formal education. Again it was suggested that instead of living in the past and in the present as a victim that I had a choice to change since I was no longer using alcohol. I remember being offended that someone would call me a victim. Today I can laugh at that, but how true it was. I had been seeing a therapist for some of my past and then present issues. She asked me to volunteer in one of her family groups, and I accepted. I fell in love with the idea of becoming a family therapist on my very first night as a volunteer. My therapist encouraged me to go forward to get the education, and of course, I put up all kinds of excuses, starting with my age, financial fear, and the biggest fear of all: fear of failure. With a lot of encouragement and trepidation I again took a small step into a new career. So at the ripe old age of 47 I went back to school and received my high school degree. I fell in love with school. I had always thought I was a terrible student. That was not true. I was a good student. Again I was being validated by others, namely teachers, and my low self-esteem began to rise. I was working as a real estate broker at this time, so I was able to financially pay for my schooling, but when I went on to get my Bachelors degree, I found it very difficult to write out that first tuition check. I actually sat there in tears because I did not yet feel good enough to spend the money on myself. Perseverance was another of the gifts I had received in my sobriety and with that and an incredible amount of emotional support I graduated with a Master's degree in Psychology at the age of 53. I then spent the next two years working as an intern in order to receive my license as a Marriage and Family Therapist. The greatest gift I learned in my schooling was that it was O.K. for me to make mistakes. I received 95% on a paper that I had written and I asked my professor (an extremely wise woman) what I had done wrong. She was able to give me this nugget: "If I could accept my mistakes and not beat myself up I would be able to learn from them." I try hard to practice that wisdom today, resulting in improved self-esteem and being good enough.

My passion for the work that I do today is just as strong as it was when I had the first thought it was possible. Early in my career I had one of the greatest opportunities of my life: I was offered the position of family therapist for a major local hospital, which was starting a 30-day treatment program for alcoholics and their families. I was given the job of developing the Family Program and then working each week for five days with multiple family members and their inpatients. In the years that I was privileged to work there I was given the gift of seeing over 1000 alcoholic patients and their families struggle on Monday morning with every issue imaginable and by Friday afternoon see in them the beginning of hope for a solution. I was also a first-hand witness of the devastation that alcohol and drugs has not only on the addict but also on family members. Today, I have been fortunate to be able to continue my work in private practice, but I am proud to say that I still volunteer at that same hospital. I have so much gratitude to that hospital, the staff and to all the families that taught me so much, for giving me the opportunity to understand in depth that this is a family disease.

As I was leaving the hospital to go into full time private practice in the mid 1980s my Higher Power rewarded me with yet another incredible gift, this was the opportunity to carry the message to the Soviet Union with several other members of Creating a Sober World (founded by Faith Strong in 1983). I now had 10 years of sobriety. We arrived in Moscow in November 1987. Gorbachev was in power and he had given permission for us to bring the Fellowship. One or two groups had preceded our group, but there was only one meeting in Moscow. There was much work to be done.

We were followed constantly by the KGB, better known as the secret police. We illegally brought in printed pages of the 12 steps and the 12 traditions. We were to see that the propaganda between the two countries had left us with the wrong opinion of people living in the USSR at that time. Controlled to the max by their government, they were not able to meet in groups nor practice any type of religion or traditions. We learned that these people had a very special kind of spirituality despite the unimaginable control they experienced.

I was to go back to the Soviet Union two more times: the last time with a team to teach sixty Latvian physicians alcoholism treatment as we practice it here in the United States. This was one of the most fearful experiences (remember the uneducated lady) and one of the most joyful experiences in my life. It was in the Soviet Union that I was finally to understand, that my physically abusive father did not have a chance with his alcoholism, he had died in England before the Fellowship reached that country. It was on my first trip to Moscow in November that I realized that the gift of sobriety for my Dad was unavailable, and how lucky I was to be handed that gift. It was there and then that I was to experience true forgiveness and be at peace. Working in the USSR with both alcoholics and al-anons, I gained many friends.

The Soviet government allowed some of these friends to come to the International Seattle Convention. I cannot even imagine what that experience was like for them, to be able to come and be free in the United States. By God's Grace I was able to be part of such an historical moment in time. I was overwhelmed and in tears when I was invited to join the Soviets in carrying their Al-Anon flag onto the convention floor. I know that there was not a dry eye in the house.

I was invited to go back to Siberia again to professionally train doctors in the western treatment of alcoholism. The year was 1992. Suddenly I was diagnosed with breast cancer and was not able to go. Instead I started cancer treatment. Because of that treatment I had to ask others for help – something that was difficult for me, but it was in asking for help that I experienced so much love and support that I was often in tears because of the gratitude I felt for this wonderful group of people that would pray for me and drop everything to walk me through this illness, physically, emotionally and spiritually. The cancer returned with a vengeance eleven years later, and it was because of my earlier experience that I was able to ask and receive that loving help one more time. Today I am healthy, sober, and eternally grateful to all the people that I have met on this blessed journey.

So what are these Glories of Sobriety? For me, I would need many more pages to let the reader know the extent of the gifts I have received. Today I know that this precious gift of sobriety has been given to me by the Grace of God and that I treasure it more than I can explain. As long as I retain that gift, I can live my life with a set of tools that helps me live an amazing life, no matter what comes my way. I know that in the painful times if I do not pick up a drink, that I will have more wisdom in seeking an appropriate solution. I hope that I have gained some humility, by allowing people to live their own lives and to be accepting of that. I am proud of my children who live good lives without my need to control and interfere. My self-esteem is good because I was taught that I am good enough. I have learned great lessons about blame, and that blame never gets me into a solution. I have freedom, friends, choices, a sense of humor and spend a whole lot of time just having fun.

Today, though my life is certainly not perfect, it is life on life's terms. So the solution for me is an enormous amount of gratitude for my sobriety, nothing more, nothing less.

Biography

Rita McCabe was born and raised in England. At the age of 14 she left school due to family circumstances. She met and married her American husband, an officer in the United States Air Force, immigrated to the United States, where they raised their family of three children. Several assignments both overseas and in different states led Rita to her ongoing passion for travel. She often travels back to England to spend time with her family. Travel is just one of Rita's interests; she also enjoys spending time with family and friends, reading, attending book clubs and going to movies. Rita has a Master's degree in Clinical Psychology and her own private practice, specializing in Addiction Therapy.

Discussion/Reflection Questions

1. How do you treat yourself if you make a mistake?

2. Where does it get you when you blame others or yourself for where your life is today?

3. How can you free yourself from self-abuse?

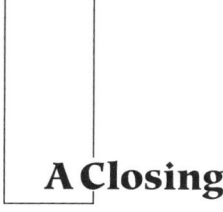

A Closing

Well, the vision has been manifested. I would like to thank our remarkable authors; our gifted, perceptive and patient editors, Barry Lyerly and Joyce Lerner; our responsible publisher, New Directions for Women in Costa Mesa, California; also, everyone who has supported and contributed to this project.

Without exception every writer was challenged by describing his or her sobriety from a different view. And, each of us can be congratulated for accepting the editors' suggestions and changes, for being willing to improve our writing and for doing it. I know too that each of us has come away from our efforts with a deeper appreciation and understanding of our sobriety and of ourselves.

Even within the diversity a common thread runs throughout the chapters: a profound commitment to a spiritual program and to being of service. Perhaps these become the foundation, the insurance for a lifelong and unshakable sobriety.

I wanted to create an open and honest book with depth, beauty, humor and joy. I think you will agree that this has been accomplished.

When feelings write our words, they move, they create, they inspire and they are authentic.

May the words in this book move you to a better place, a better life – a better way.

With Love,

—Faith Strong
Editor

"I do not know what your destiny will be, but one thing I do know: the only ones among you who will be really happy are those who have sought and found how to serve."

Dr. Albert Schweitzer